Immediate Life Support

6th Edition, November 2025

ILS

Immediate Life Support
6th Edition, November 2025

ISBN 978-1-903812-43-3

Published by © Resuscitation Council UK
1st Floor, 60–62 Margaret Street, London, W1W 8TF
Tel: 020 7388 4678 email: enquiries@resus.org.uk www.resus.org.uk

Printed by All About Print
Tel: 020 7205 4022 email: hello@allaboutprint.co.uk www.allaboutprint.co.uk
Printed on responsibly sourced environmentally friendly paper made with elemental chlorine free fibre from legal and sustainably managed forests.

Photographs © Resuscitation Council UK.
Photography by Ed Tyler, Ashley Prytherch and Mike Scott
Chain of Prevention © Gary Smith
Chain of Survival © European Resuscitation Council
ECGs © Oliver Meyer
Electrical conduction of the heart (Figure 8.4) © LifeART image (1989–2001) Wolters Kluwer Health, Inc. Lippincott Williams & Wilkins. All rights reserved.

Design and artwork by Fruition London
www.fruitionlondon.com

The Resuscitation Council UK guidelines are adapted from the European Resuscitation Council guidelines. The UK guidelines are consistent with the European guidelines but include minor modifications to reflect the needs of the National Health Service.

The NCAA is the national, comparative clinical audit of in-hospital cardiac arrests for hospitals in the UK and Ireland. NCAA is supported by Resuscitation Council UK and Intensive Care National Audit & Research Centre (ICNARC). We thank all the staff at hospitals participating in the NCAA. For more information on the representativeness and quality of these data, please contact ICNARC.

This Immediate Life Support manual forms part of the resources for the Resuscitation Council UK course, which is delivered in accredited course centres throughout the UK.

MIX
Supporting responsible forestry
FSC® C013417
www.fsc.org

CARBON BALANCED PAPER
www.carbonbalancedpaper.com
CBP032574

Acknowledgements

We thank the Nuffield Hospital, Guildford, for the use of their facilities, and the Royal Surrey NHS Foundation Trust, particularly the Resuscitation Department, for their assistance with photography. We also thank the London Ambulance Service for the use of their facilities and the support of their team during photography, and Lifecast Body Simulation for the loan of manikins. Our gratitude extends to all the instructors who generously gave their time to take part in the photography shoot.

We are grateful to Oliver Meyer for the digital preparation of the 12-lead ECGs and rhythm strips. We also thank Ed Tyler, Ashley Prytherch and Mike Scott for their work on the photography, and Kerstin Rivett for the digital preparation of the manual.

The Hot Debrief STOP-5 tool is reproduced with the kind permission of Dr Craig Walker, on behalf of Edinburgh Emergency Medicine and The Scottish Centre for Simulation & Clinical Human Factors.

Commitment to inclusive language

The language and assessment techniques in this manual are benchmarked against current NHS materials and informed by specialist Equity, Equality, Diversity and Inclusivity (EEDI) organisations with whom we consult.

We recognise that language in the equity space evolves rapidly, and some terms used here may become outdated during the lifespan of this manual. We will strive to update the content as soon as practicable to reflect current best practice.

Editors

Joyce Yeung
Adam Benson Clarke
Michael Bradfield
Isabelle Hamilton-Bower
Victoria Wragg

Contributors

Catherine Baldock
Adam Benson Clarke
Michael Bradfield
Matthew Cordingly
Mandy Chalk
Keith Chaplin
Ron Daniels
Robin Davies
Charles Deakin
Richard Field
Catriona Fleming
James Fullerton
David Gabbott
Holly Grant
Carl Gwinnutt
Isabelle Hamilton-Bower
Sue Hampshire
Ian Hanson
Dan Higgins
Justin Honey Jones
Joanna Lawrence
Emily Le-Gallienne
Bernadette Lee
Andrew Lockey
Kevin Mackie
Paul Marlow
Mary Murphy
Jerry Nolan
Gavin Perkins
David Pitcher
Susanna Price
Emily Reynolds
Mike Scott
Fiona Smith
Gary Smith
Jasmeet Soar
Stephen Williams
Victoria Wragg
Joyce Yeung

Contents

Contents

Notes

Glossary

Abbreviation	In full
A	amperes
ABCDE	refers to the Airway, Breathing, Circulation, Disability, Exposure assessment
AED	automated external defibrillator
AMI	acute myocardial infarction
CPR	cardiopulmonary resuscitation – this refers to chest compressions and ventilations
ECG	electrocardiogram
EWS	early warning score
ICNARC	Intensive Care National Audit & Research Centre
IV	intravenous
IO	intraosseous
NCAA	National Cardiac Arrest Audit
NEWS	national early warning score
NSTE ACS	non-ST-segment-elevation acute coronary syndromes
NSTEMI	non-ST-elevation myocardial infarction
PEA	pulseless electrical activity
POCUS	point of care ultra sound
ReSPECT	Recommended Summary Plan for Emergency Care and Treatment
ROSC	return of spontaneous circulation
RSVP	reason, story, vital signs, plan
SBARD	Situation, Background, Assessment, Recommendation, Decision
SCD	sudden cardiac death
Shockable rhythm	refers to cardiac arrest rhythms that can be treated with CPR and a defibrillator
UA	unstable angina
VF	ventricular fibrillation – VF is a shockable cardiac arrest rhythm
VT	ventricular tachycardia
pVT	pulseless ventricular tachycardia – pVT is a shockable cardiac arrest rhythm
VF/pVT	VF or pulseless VT – these are both shockable cardiac arrest rhythms

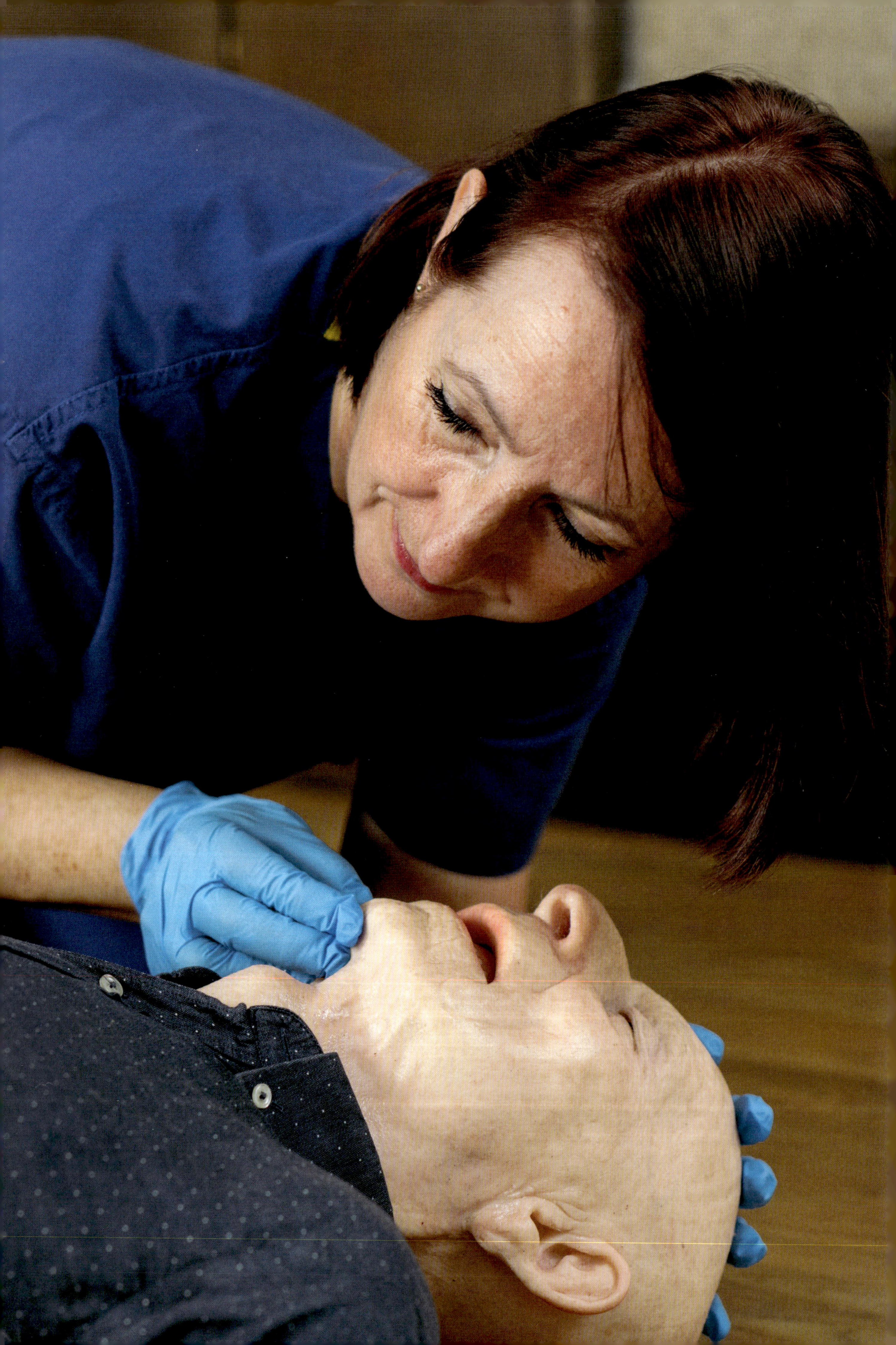

01 Introduction to immediate life support

In this chapter

About the Immediate Life Support course

Improving patient outcomes

Evidence-based guidelines

Quality standards

Measuring patient outcomes

The learning outcomes will enable you to:

Use the manual to support your development as an ILS provider

Understand the value of adopting evidence-informed guidelines and setting quality standards to improve patient outcomes from cardiac arrest

Understand the importance of measuring patient outcomes and safety incident reporting to improve care

Aim of the course

Many cardiac arrests are preventable. Resuscitation Council UK's (RCUK) Immediate Life Support (ILS) course provides you with essential knowledge and skills to treat adults in cardiac arrest before and after the arrival of the emergency response team.

The ILS course will show you how to recognise and initiate appropriate treatment of the deteriorating patient using the Airway, Breathing, Circulation, Disability, Exposure (ABCDE) assessment. If cardiac arrest does occur, the skills taught on the ILS course are those that are most likely used to resuscitate the patient.

A B C D E

How to use the course manual

This evidence-informed manual is designed to be used before, during and after the course. The contents of this manual are essential reading to help your learning. The manual includes questions throughout to help you assess your understanding of each chapter. The additional reading will help further your knowledge and understanding to better prepare you when applying your skills in practice.

How to use the e-learning

The online eILS modules will complement your learning. There are a range of interactive activities which can be accessed before your face-to-face training.

Improving patient outcomes from deterioration and cardiac arrest

High-quality care is safe, effective, patient-centred, timely, efficient and equitable. Emergency response teams, including ILS providers, should ensure they deliver high-quality care to improve the treatment and outcomes of deteriorating patients and patients in cardiac arrest. Interventions to improve patient outcomes are described below.

Figure 1.1 Delivery of high quality care

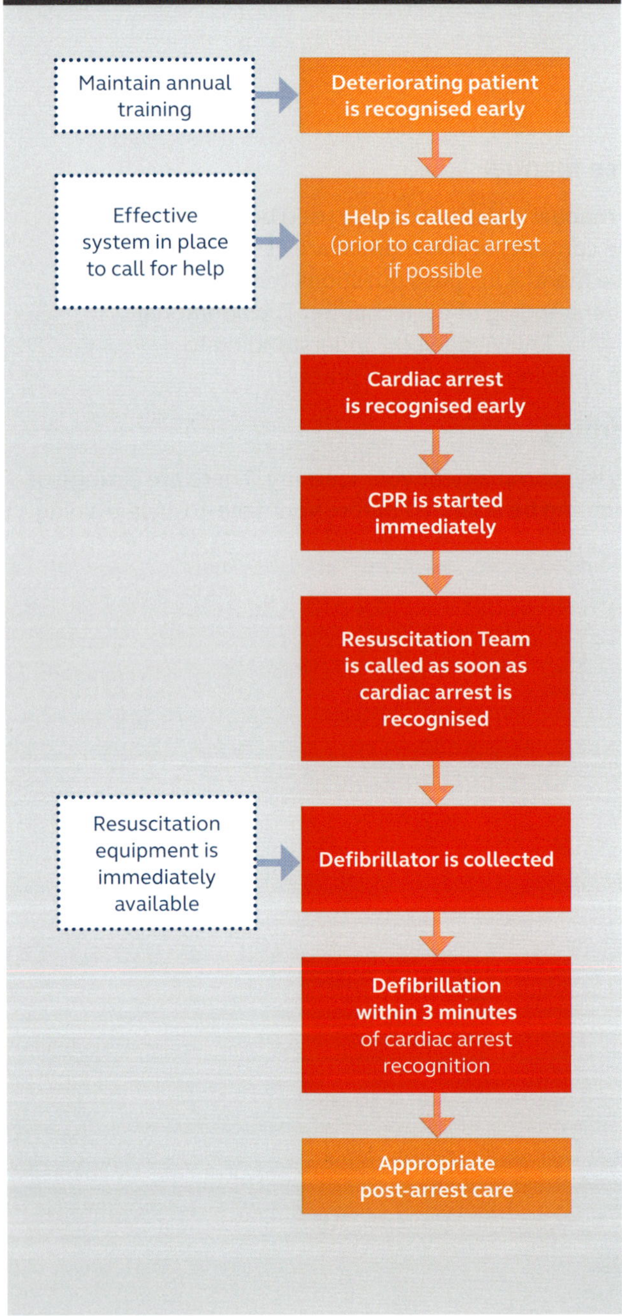

Evidence-informed guidelines

Improving outcomes from cardiac arrest depends on the implementation of evidence-based guidelines. Immediate Life Support is consistent with the current Resuscitation Council UK Guidelines. The guidelines are based on:

- Systematic reviews with grading of the quality of evidence and strength of recommendations.
- The involvement of stakeholders, including members of the public and cardiac arrest survivors, so that their values and preferences can be considered in guidelines.

The current Resuscitation Council UK Guidelines for cardiopulmonary resuscitation can be found at (www.resus.org.uk).

Quality standards

Hospitals and healthcare settings are obliged to provide a high-quality resuscitation service that ensures staff are trained according to their expected roles. The same core standards apply to all healthcare settings to ensure that:

- The deteriorating patient is recognised early, and there is an effective system to summon help in order to prevent cardiac arrest.
- Cardiac arrest is recognised early, and cardiopulmonary resuscitation (CPR) is started immediately.
- Emergency assistance is summoned immediately, as soon as cardiac arrest is recognised, if help has not been summoned.
- Defibrillation, if appropriate, is attempted within 3 minutes of identifying cardiac arrest.
- Appropriate post-arrest care is received by those who are resuscitated successfully. This includes safe transfer.
- Implementation of standards is measured continually, and processes are in place to deal with any problems identified.
- Staff receive at least annual training and updates in CPR, based on their expected roles.
- Staff understand decisions relating to CPR.
- Appropriate equipment is immediately available for resuscitation.

Resuscitation Council UK Quality Standards for cardiopulmonary resuscitation practice and training provide further detailed information. These standards include suggested equipment lists for different health care settings.

Measuring patient outcomes

Continuous measurement of compliance with processes and patient outcomes at both national and local levels provides information on the impact of changes in practice, identifies areas for improvement, and enables comparison of outcomes between different organisations. Uniform definitions for collecting data for cardiac arrest exist.

The National Cardiac Arrest Audit (NCAA) is an ongoing, national, comparative outcome audit of in-hospital cardiac arrests. It is a joint initiative between Resuscitation Council UK and the Intensive Care National Audit & Research Centre (ICNARC). It is open to all acute hospitals in the UK and Ireland. The audit monitors and reports on the incidence of and outcome from in-hospital cardiac arrest to inform practice and policy. It aims to identify and foster improvements in the prevention, care delivery and outcomes from cardiac arrest.

Data are collected according to standardised definitions and entered onto the NCAA secure web-based system. Once data are validated, hospitals are provided with activity reports and risk-adjusted comparative reports, allowing comparisons to be made not only within, but also between, hospitals locally, nationally, and internationally. In 2023–24, the overall survival of adult in-hospital cardiac arrest to discharge was 25.8%.

The National Out-of-Hospital Cardiac Arrest Outcomes project measures patient, process, and outcome variables related to out-of-hospital cardiac arrest in the UK. The project is run in collaboration with the National Ambulance Service Medical Directors' Group, with support from the British Heart Foundation, Resuscitation Council UK, and the University of Warwick. The project is designed to measure the epidemiology and outcomes of cardiac arrest and to serve as a national resource for continuous quality improvement initiatives for cardiac arrest. Among those in whom resuscitation is attempted, 30% initially achieve a return of spontaneous circulation (ROSC), but only 9% survive to go home from the hospital.

My key take-home messages from this chapter are:

01 SUMMARY LEARNING

Evidence-based high-quality care can improve treatment and outcomes of deteriorating patients and patients in cardiac arrest.

Further reading

National Out-of-Hospital Cardiac Arrest Outcomes Project. www.warwick.ac.uk/ohcao

Greif R, Perkins GD, Gräsner JT, et al. European Resuscitation Council Guidelines 2025: Executive summary. Resuscitation. 2025. In print.

Intensive Care National Audit & Research Centre (2024) National Cardiac Arrest Audit: Summary Statistics 2022–23. London: ICNARC. Available at: https://www.icnarc.org/wp-content/uploads/2024/05/NCAA-Summary-Statistics-2022-23.pdf.pdf (Accessed: 10 July 2025).

Nabecker S, de Raad T, Conaghan P, et al. European Resuscitation Council Guidelines 2025: Education of Resuscitation. Resuscitation. 2025. In print.

Perkins GD, Graesner JT, Semeraro F, Olasveengen T, Soar J, Lott C, Van de Voorde P, Madar J, Zideman D, Mentzelopoulos S, Bossaert L, Greif R, Monsieurs K, Svasvasdottir H and Nolan JP. European Resuscitation Council Guidelines 2021–Executive summary. Resuscitation. 2021;161.

Nolan JP, Soar J, Smith GB, et al. Incidence and outcome of in-hospital cardiac arrest in the United Kingdom National Cardiac Arrest Audit. Resuscitation 2014;85:987-92.

Olasveengen TM, Semeraro F, Ristagno G, Castren M, Handley A, Kuzovlev A, Monsieurs KG, Raffay V, Smyth M, Soar J, Svavarsdottir H and Perkins GD. European Resuscitation Council Guidelines 2021: Basic Life Support. Resuscitation. 2021;161.

Resuscitation Council UK. Quality standards for cardiopulmonary resuscitation and training. https://www.resus.org.uk/library/ quality-standards-cpr

Semeraro F, Schnaubelt S, Olasveengen TM, et al. European Resuscitation Council Guidelines 2025: Systems Saving Lives. Resuscitation. 2025. In print.

Soar J, Carli P, Couper K, Deakin CD, Djarv T, Lott C, Olasveengen TM, Paal P, Pellis T, Perkins GD, Sandroni C, Nolan JP. European Resuscitation Council Guidelines 2021: Advanced Life Support. Resuscitation. 2021;161.

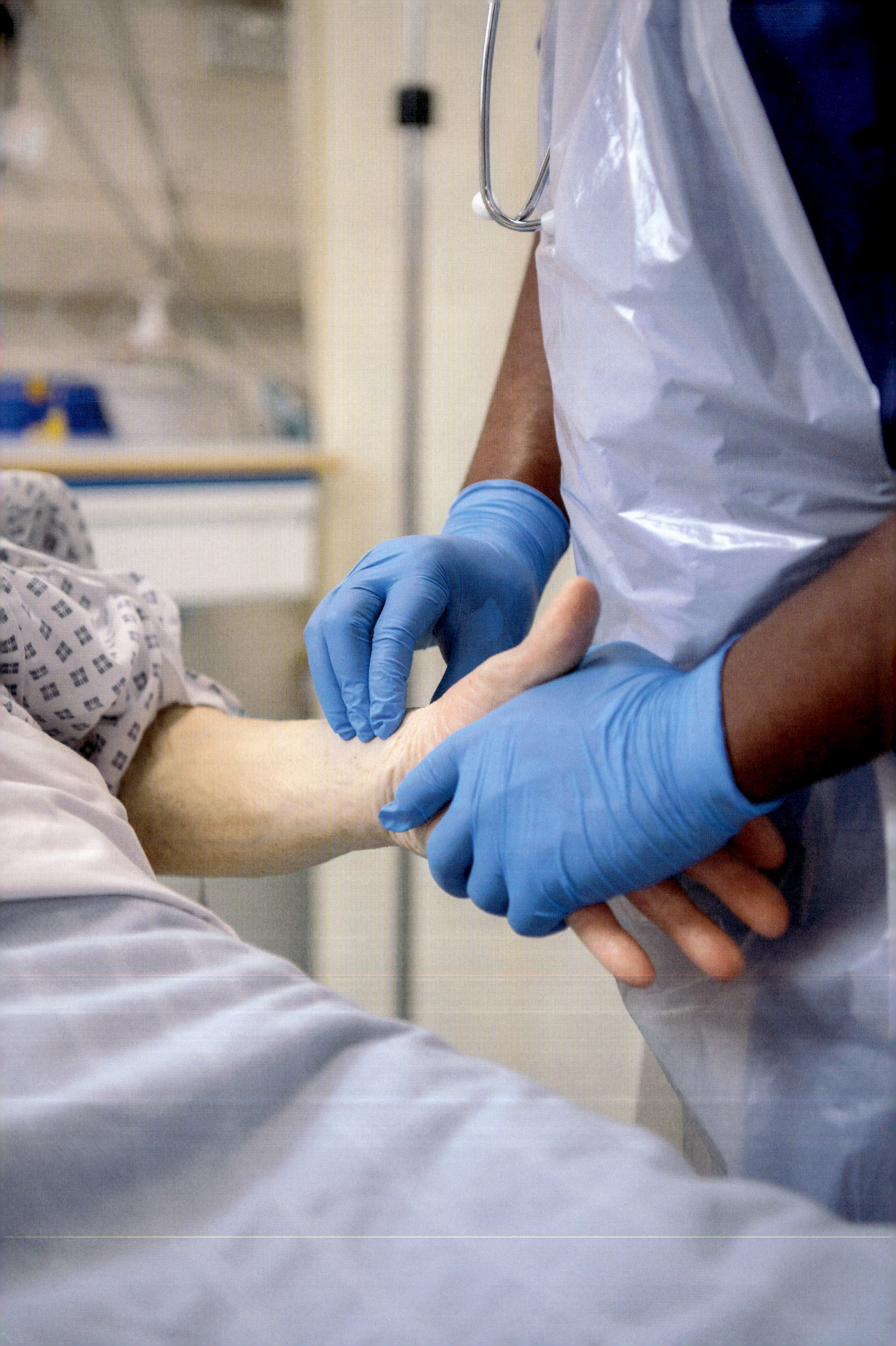

02 Recognising the deterioating patient

In this chapter

Prevention of cardiac arrest: the Chain of Prevention

Recognising the deteriorating patient

Response to critical illness

Causes of deterioration and cardiac arrest

The ABCDE assessment

Look, listen and feel

The learning outcomes will enable you to:

Understand the importance of early recognition of the deteriorating patient

Consider the relevant causes of cardiac arrest in adults

Identify and treat patients at risk of cardiac arrest using the Airway, Breathing, Circulation, Disability, Exposure (ABCDE) assessment

Introduction

Early recognition of a deteriorating patient and prevention of cardiac arrest are the first link in the Chain of Survival (Chapter 3). Once cardiac arrest occurs, 25.8% of all patients having an in-hospital cardiac arrest survive to go home. Prevention of cardiac arrest in a clinical setting requires staff education, monitoring of patients, recognition of patient deterioration, a system to call for help, and an effective response.

Survival after in-hospital cardiac arrest is more likely if the arrest is witnessed and monitored, the rhythm is a shockable rhythm with the primary cause of myocardial ischaemia, and the patient is defibrillated immediately.

Most in-hospital cardiac arrests are not sudden or unpredictable events: in up to 80% of cases, there is deterioration in clinical signs during the few hours before cardiac arrest.

These patients often have slow and progressive physiological deterioration, particularly hypoxia and hypotension (i.e. Airway, Breathing, and Circulation problems) that is unnoticed by staff, or is recognised but not appropriately managed.

The presenting cardiac arrest rhythms in this group were shockable (VF/pVT) in 18.1% and non-shockable (asystole (19.9%) or pulseless electrical activity (52%) in 71.9% of cases, and rates of survival to hospital discharge associated with these rhythms were 52.9% for shockable rhythms, and 17.1% and 11.5% for PEA and asystole respectively.

Early recognition and effective treatment of the deteriorating patient might prevent cardiac arrest, death or an unanticipated admission to the intensive care unit (ICU). Early recognition will also help to identify individuals for whom cardiopulmonary resuscitation (CPR) is not appropriate or who do not wish to be resuscitated (Chapter 5).

Much of this chapter is based on the deteriorating patient in the hospital setting. However, the same basic principles apply to the care of the deteriorating patient in the out-of-hospital setting.

Figure 2.1 Early recognition: the Chain of Prevention

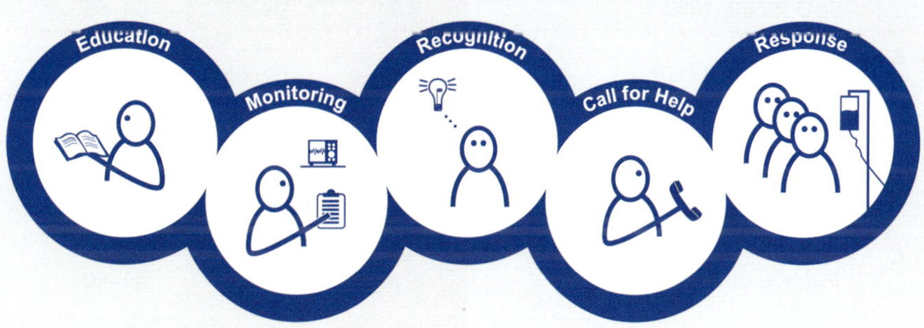

Prevention of cardiac arrest: The Chain of Prevention

The Chain of Prevention (Figure 2.1) can help staff in clinical settings structure care processes to prevent and detect patient deterioration and cardiac arrest. There are five links in the chain:

1. Education

Education should include how to observe patients, interpretation of observed signs and signs of deterioration. It should also include the use of the ABCDE assessment, simple skills to prevent further deterioration until help arrives and the rationale for activating rapid response systems.

2. Monitoring

Monitoring and patient assessment require the measurement and recording of vital signs, and accurate documentation.

3. Recognition

Recognition encompasses the tools available to identify patients in need of additional monitoring or intervention, including suitably designed vital signs charts and sets of predetermined 'calling criteria' to 'flag' the need to escalate monitoring or to call for more expert help.

4. Call for help

Call for help protocols for summoning a response to a deteriorating patient should be universally known and understood, unambiguous and mandated. All staff in clinical settings should be empowered to call for help.

A call for help should use a structured communication tool such as **SBARD** (Situation, Background, Assessment, Recommendation, Decision) or **RSVP** (Reason, Story, Vital signs, Plan).

5. Response

Clinicians who rapidly respond to a deteriorating patient should have appropriate knowledge, skills and experience. Rapid response systems should be in place (e.g. from an emergency response team, critical care outreach team or resuscitation team).

Recognising the deteriorating patient

In general, the clinical signs of critical illness are similar whatever the underlying cause because they reflect failing respiratory, cardiovascular, and neurological systems (i.e. ABCDE problems, see below). To help early detection of deteriorating patients, many clinical settings use early warning scores (EWS). EWS systems allocate points to measurements of routine vital signs based on their deviation from an agreed 'normal' range.

The weighted score of one or more vital signs, or the total EWS, indicates the level of intervention required (e.g. increased frequency of vital signs monitoring, or the need to call for further help). In the UK, the National Early Warning Score 2 (**NEWS2**) is recommended (Table 2.1) for all non-pregnant patients over the age of 16 years.

The EWS is dynamic and change over time and the frequency of observations should be increased to track improvement or deterioration in a patient's condition. If it is clear a patient is deteriorating, call for help early rather than wait for the patient to reach a specific score.

Table 2.1 National Early Warning Score 2 (NEWS2)

Physiological parameter		Score						
		3	2	1	0	1	2	3
A & B	Respiration rate (per minute)	≤ 8		9–11	12–20		21–24	≥ 25
	SpO_2 Scale 1 (%)	≤ 91	92–93	94–95	≥ 96			
	SpO_2 Scale 2 (%)*	≤ 83	84–85	86–87	88–92 ≥ 93 on air	93–94 on oxygen	95–96 on oxygen	≥ 97 on oxygen
	Air or oxygen?		Oxygen		Air			
C	Systolic blood pressure (mmHg)	≤ 90	91–100	101–110	111–219			≥ 220
	Pulse (per minute)	≤ 40		41–50	51–90	91–110	111–130	≥ 131
D	Consciousness**				Alert			Confusion VPU
E	Temperature (°C)	≤ 35.0		35.1–36.0	36.1–38.0	38.1–39.0	≥ 39.1	

* Use Scale 2 if target range is 88–92% (e.g. in hypercapnic respiratory failure).

** Score for new onset confusion, no score if chronic confusion.

The patient's total EWS is calculated as the sum of physiological parameters as seen in Table 2.1. An increased score indicates an increased risk of deterioration and death. There should be a graded response to scores according to local procedures. An example of escalation plan is shown in Table 2.2.

Clinician concern may also be an important predictor of patient deterioration (Figure 2.2). Even when a more senior clinician is alerted to a patient's abnormal physiology, there is often delay in attending to the patient or referring to higher levels of care.

Response to critical illness

The traditional response to cardiac arrest is reactive: the name 'resuscitation team' implies that it will be called only after a cardiac arrest has occurred.

In many hospitals, the resuscitation team has been incorporated into rapid response systems (e.g. rapid response team, critical care outreach team, medical emergency team (MET)). These teams can be activated according to the patient's EWS (see above) or according to specific calling criteria.

For example, the MET typically comprises medical and nursing staff from intensive care and acute medicine and responds to specific calling criteria and cardiac arrests. Any member of the healthcare team, and in some cases the patient or their relatives, can initiate a MET call. Early involvement of the MET may reduce cardiac arrests, deaths and unanticipated ICU admissions, and may facilitate anticipatory care discussions e.g. ReSPECT or do not attempt cardiopulmonary resuscitation (DNACPR).

Figure 2.2 Healthcare professional assessing a sick patient

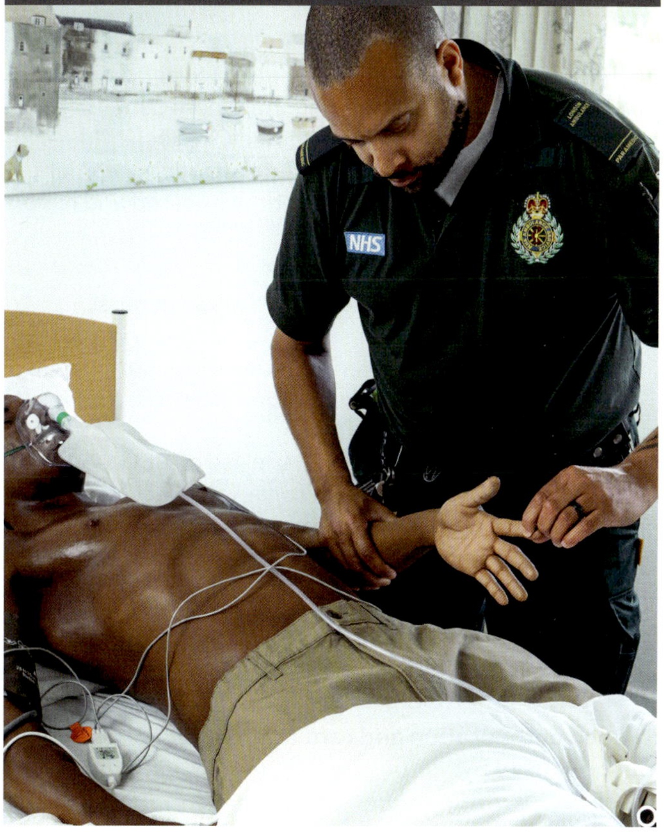

The rapid response system can vary between organisations. Clinicians should be familiar with which rapid response system within your organisation. Critically ill patients should be admitted to a critical care area (e.g. ICU, high dependency unit (HDU), or resuscitation room). These areas are staffed by healthcare professionals experienced in advanced resuscitation and critical care skills.

Table 2.2 Escalation protocol based on early warning score

NEW score	Frequency of monitoring	Clinical response
0	**Minimum 12 hourly**	Continue routine NEWS2 monitoring.
Total 1–4	**Minimum 4–6 hourly**	Inform registered nurse, who must assess the patient. Registered nurse decides whether increased frequency of monitoring and/or escalation of care is required.
3 in single parameter	**Minimum 1 hourly**	Registered nurse to inform medical team caring for the patient, who will review and decide whether escalation of care is necessary.
Total 5 or 6: Urgent response threshold	**Minimum 1 hourly**	Registered nurse to immediately inform the medical team caring for the patient. Registered nurse to request urgent assessment by a clinician or team with core competencies in the care of acutely ill patients. Provide clinical care in an environment with monitoring facilities.
Total 7 or more: Emergency response threshold	**Continuous monitoring of vital signs**	Registered nurse to immediately inform the medical team caring for the patient – this should be at least at specialist registrar level. Emergency assessment by a team with critical care competencies, including practitioner(s) with advanced airway management skills. Consider transfer of care to a level 2 or 3 clinical care facility i.e. higher-dependency unit or ICU. Clinical care in an environment with monitoring facilities.

In hospitals, staffing tends to be at its lowest during the night and at weekends. This influences patient monitoring, treatment and outcomes. In-hospital cardiac arrests occurring in the late afternoon, at night or at weekends are more often non-witnessed and have a lower survival rate.

Patients discharged at night from ICUs to general wards have an increased risk of ICU readmission and in-hospital death compared with those discharged during the day and those discharged to HDUs.

In out-of-hospital environments, the use of NEWS2 can support discharge, referral and conveyance decisions and should be handed over to the receiving team at hospital. Patients with a high NEWS2 score on initial assessment should be monitored carefully for deterioration during transfer.

Causes of deterioration and cardiac arrest

Sudden deterioration and cardiac arrest can be caused by:

- **Airway, and/or**
- **Breathing, and/or**
- **Circulation problems.**

A = Airway obstruction

Airway obstruction can be complete or partial.

Complete airway obstruction rapidly causes cardiac arrest.

Partial obstruction often precedes complete obstruction. Partial airway obstruction can cause cerebral or pulmonary oedema, exhaustion, secondary apnoea, hypoxic brain injury, and eventually cardiac arrest.

For a detailed review of airway management see Chapter 9.

Causes of airway obstruction

- Blockage in airway: blood, secretions, vomitus, foreign body (dislodged teeth, food).
- Infection and oedema: direct trauma to face or throat, epiglottitis, pharyngeal swelling.
- Narrowing of airway: laryngospasm, bronchospasm.
- Central nervous system depression: this may cause loss of airway patency and protective reflexes. Causes include head injury and intracerebral disease, hypercapnia, the depressant effect of metabolic disorders (e.g. hypoglycaemia in diabetic patients), and drugs (e.g. alcohol, opioids and general anaesthetic).

Figure 2.3 Response to deteriorating patient

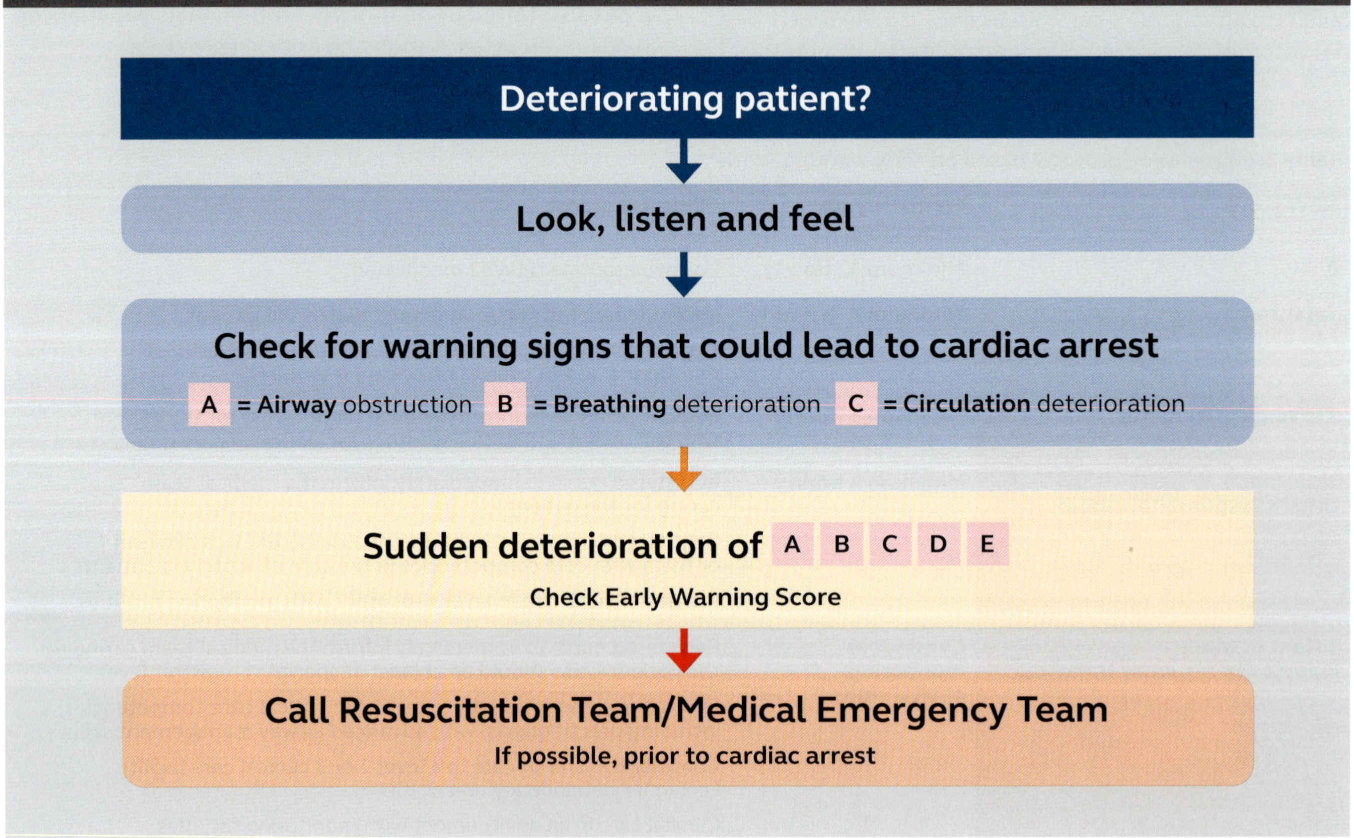

Recognition of airway obstruction

The following signs may be seen and are discussed in more detail in Chapter 9.

- A conscious patient will complain of difficulty in breathing.
- Choking.
- Noisy breathing is seen in partial airway obstruction.
- Complete airway obstruction is silent and there is no air movement at the patient's mouth. Any respiratory movements are usually strenuous.
- The accessory muscles of respiration will be involved, causing a 'see-saw' or 'rocking-horse' pattern of chest and abdominal movement: the chest is drawn in and the abdomen expands on inspiration, and the opposite occurs on expiration.

Treatment of airway obstruction (See page 21)

- The priority is to ensure that the airway remains patent. Treat any problem that places the airway at risk; for example, use suction to remove any blood and gastric contents from the airway and, unless contraindicated, turn the patient on their side.
- Administer high-flow oxygen as soon as possible to achieve an oxygen saturation level (SpO_2) of 94–98% or 88–92% in patients with hypercapnic respiratory failure.
- Assume actual or impending airway obstruction in anyone with a depressed level of consciousness, regardless of cause.
- Take steps to safeguard the airway and prevent further complications such as aspiration of gastric contents. This may involve positioning the patient on their side or with a head-up tilt.
- Airway patency may be improved by simple airway opening manoeuvres such as head tilt/chin lift or jaw thrust. Adjuncts such as nasopharyngeal airways, oropharyngeal airways, or supraglottic airway devices may also be used if available.
- Tracheal intubation by an airway expert may be required.
- Consider insertion of a nasogastric tube to empty the stomach.

B = Breathing problems

Causes of breathing problems

Breathing inadequacy may be acute or chronic. It may be continuous or intermittent, and severe enough to cause the person to stop breathing (apnoea or respiratory arrest). This will rapidly lead to a secondary cardiac arrest if not treated.

Respiratory arrest often arises from a combination of factors. In a patient with chronic respiratory inadequacy, a chest infection, muscle weakness, or fractured ribs may lead to exhaustion, further depressing respiratory function. If breathing is insufficient to oxygenate the blood adequately, lack of oxygen to the vital organs will lead to loss of consciousness and eventually cardiac arrest.

Respiratory drive

Central nervous system depression can decrease or abolish respiratory drive. The causes are the same as those for airway obstruction from central nervous system depression.

Respiratory effort

The main respiratory muscles are the diaphragm and intercostal muscles. The latter are innervated at the level of their respective ribs and may be paralysed by a spinal cord lesion above this level. The innervation of the diaphragm is derived from the third, fourth and fifth segment of the cervical spinal cord. Spontaneous breathing cannot occur with severe cervical cord damage above this level.

Inadequate respiratory effort, caused by muscle weakness or nerve damage, occurs with many diseases (e.g. myasthenia gravis, Guillain-Barré syndrome, and multiple sclerosis). Chronic malnourishment and severe long-term illness may also contribute to generalised weakness.

Breathing can also be impaired with restrictive chest wall abnormalities such as kyphoscoliosis. Pain from fractured ribs or sternum will prevent deep breaths and coughing.

Lung disorders

Severe lung disease will impair gas exchange. Causes include infection, exacerbation of chronic obstructive pulmonary disease (COPD), asthma, pulmonary embolism (PE), lung contusion, acute respiratory distress syndrome (ARDS) and pulmonary oedema. Lung function is also impaired by a pneumothorax or haemothorax. A tension pneumothorax impairs gas exchange and reduces venous return to the heart causing a decrease in cardiac output and is a medical emergency.

Recognition of breathing problems

- A conscious patient will complain of shortness of breath and be distressed.
- The history and examination will usually indicate the underlying cause.
- Hypoxaemia and hypercapnia can cause irritability, confusion, lethargy and depressed consciousness.
- Cyanosis is a late sign.

A high respiratory rate (> 25 min^{-1}) is a useful, simple indicator of breathing problems.

Pulse oximetry is an easy, non-invasive measure of the adequacy of oxygenation (Chapter 9).

However, it is not a reliable indicator of ventilation, and an arterial blood gas sample is necessary to obtain values for arterial carbon dioxide tension ($PaCO_2$) and pH.

A rising $PaCO_2$ and a decrease in pH are often late signs in a patient with severe respiratory problems.

Treatment of breathing problems (See page 21)

- Give oxygen to all acutely ill hypoxic patients and treat the underlying cause. Give oxygen at 15 L min^{-1} using a high-concentration reservoir mask.
- Once oxygen saturation can be measured reliably, change the oxygen mask and aim for a SpO_2 in the range of 94–98%, or 88–92% for hypercapnic (type II) respiratory failure.
- Give early intravenous (IV) antibiotics to a patient with a severe pneumonia or start a bronchodilator (salbutamol nebulisers) and steroid treatment for a patient with severe asthma.
- Patients who are having difficulty breathing or are becoming tired will need help with their breathing.
- Non-invasive ventilation using a face mask or high-flow nasal cannula can be useful in preventing the need for tracheal intubation and ventilation.
- It is best to call for expert help early for patients who cannot breathe adequately, as ICU admission for sedation, tracheal intubation, and controlled ventilation may be needed.

C = Circulation problems

Causes of circulation problems

Circulation problems can be caused by primary heart disease or by heart abnormalities secondary to other problems. In acutely ill patients, circulation problems are most commonly caused by hypovolaemia. The heart may stop suddenly or may produce an inadequate cardiac output before stopping.

Primary heart problems

Sudden cardiac arrest is most commonly caused by an arrhythmia secondary to an acute coronary syndrome – see below. The most common initial cardiac arrest rhythm is ventricular fibrillation (VF).

Acute coronary syndromes

Acute coronary syndromes (ACS) usually present with chest pain or discomfort resulting from myocardial ischaemia. The distinct categories are distinguished initially by the presence or absence of ST-segment elevation on a 12-lead ECG and, in those without ST-segment elevation, by the presence or absence of a raised blood troponin concentration suggesting myocardial injury:

- ST-segment-elevation myocardial infarction (STEMI)
- Non-ST-segment-elevation acute coronary syndromes (NSTE ACS)
  - Non-ST-segment-elevation myocardial infarction (NSTEMI)
  - Unstable angina (UA).

Recognition of acute coronary syndromes

- Acute myocardial infarction (AMI) typically presents with chest pain that is felt as a heaviness or tightness or indigestion-like discomfort in the chest. The pain or discomfort often radiates into the neck or throat, into one or both arms (more commonly the left), and into the back or into the epigastrium. Some patients experience the discomfort more in one of these areas than in the chest. This may vary between patients.
- Sometimes discomfort is accompanied by belching, which can be misinterpreted as evidence of indigestion as the cause. A history of sustained (i.e. 20–30 minutes or more) acute chest pain typical of AMI, with acute ST-segment elevation on a 12-lead ECG, is the basis for a diagnosis of STEMI.
- Some patients present with chest pain suggestive of AMI and less specific ECG abnormalities, such as ST-segment depression or T wave inversion.

- A history suggestive of ACS and laboratory tests showing substantial release of troponin indicates that myocardial damage has occurred. This is referred to as NSTEMI.
- Consider unstable angina when there is an unprovoked and prolonged episode of chest pain, raising suspicion of AMI but without definite ECG or laboratory evidence of AMI.

People with chest pain need urgent medical attention. Out of hospital they should dial 999 and call an ambulance. If they have an ACS they are at high risk of cardiac arrest and sudden cardiac death (SCD).

Initial treatment of acute coronary syndromes

Patients with an ACS should be closely monitored. Immediate treatment for ACS comprises:

- Aspirin 300 mg orally, crushed or chewed, as soon as possible
- Sublingual glyceryl trinitrate (spray or tablet) unless the patient is hypotensive
- Oxygen if the patient is hypoxic (saturation < 94% on air), titrated to target saturation of 94–98%. In the presence of hypercapnic respiratory failure, aim for 88–92%
- Pain relief with IV opiate analgesia (morphine) with an anti-emetic. The dose of morphine should be titrated to control symptoms whilst avoiding sedation and respiratory depression
- Urgent referral to a cardiologist for further treatment.

Sudden cardiac death (SCD)

Coronary artery disease is the most common cause of SCD. Non-ischaemic cardiomyopathy and valvular disease account for some other SCD events. A small percentage of SCDs are caused by inherited abnormalities (e.g. long and short QT syndromes, Brugada syndrome, hypertrophic cardiomyopathy, arrhythmogenic right ventricular cardiomyopathy), and congenital heart disease.

In patients with a known diagnosis of cardiac disease, syncope (with or without preceding symptoms – particularly if recent or recurrent) is an independent risk factor for increased risk of death. Apparently healthy children and young adults who have SCD can also have signs and symptoms (e.g. syncope/pre-syncope, chest pain, palpitation, heart murmur) that should alert healthcare professionals to seek expert help to prevent cardiac arrest.

Assessment in a clinic specialising in the care of those at risk for SCD is recommended in family members of young people with SCD. It should also be considered in those with a known cardiac disorder resulting in an increased risk of SCD. (www.nice.org.uk/guidance/cg109).

Secondary heart problems

The heart is affected by changes elsewhere in the body. For example, cardiac arrest will occur rapidly following asphyxia from airway obstruction or apnoea, or after acute severe blood loss. Severe hypoxia and anaemia, hypothermia, hypovolaemia and severe septic shock will also impair cardiac function and can lead to cardiac arrest.

Recognition of secondary heart problems

- The signs and symptoms of cardiac disease include chest pain, shortness of breath, syncope, tachycardia, bradycardia, tachypnoea (high respiratory rate), hypotension, poor peripheral perfusion (prolonged capillary refill time), altered mental state, and oliguria (low urine output).
- Most SCDs occur in people with pre-existing cardiac disease, which may have been unrecognised. Asymptomatic or silent cardiac disease includes hypertensive heart disease, aortic valve disease, cardiomyopathy, myocarditis, and coronary disease.

Treatment of secondary heart problems

Treat the underlying cause of circulatory failure. In many sick patients, this means giving oxygen to correct hypoxaemia and intravenous fluids to correct hypovolaemia.

Figure 2.4 Circulation – pulse assessment

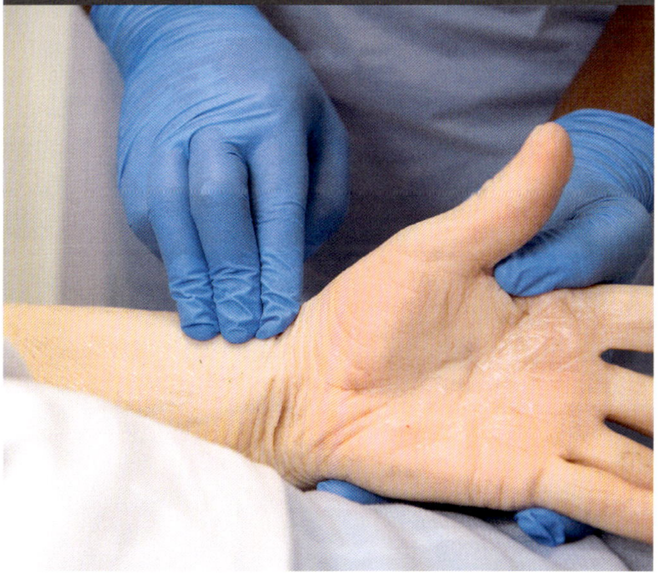

The A B C D E assessment

Underlying principles of the ABCDE assessment

The approach to all deteriorating or critically ill patients is the same. The underlying principles are:

1. **Use the Airway, Breathing, Circulation, Disability, Exposure assessment** to assess and treat the patient. The detail of your assessment and which treatments you administer will depend on your role, clinical knowledge and skills.
2. **Treat life-threatening problems** before moving to the next part of the assessment.
3. **Do a complete initial assessment** and reassess regularly for changes and effects of treatment.
4. **Recognise when you need extra help.** Call for help early.
5. **Use all team members.** This enables several interventions (e.g. assessment, attaching monitors, intravenous access) to be undertaken simultaneously.
6. **Monitor the vital signs early.** Attach a pulse oximeter, ECG monitor and a non-invasive blood pressure monitor to all critically ill patients, as soon as possible.
7. **Communicate effectively** – use **SBARD** or **RSVP** (Chapter 4).
8. **The aim is to assess the patient and give initial treatment to stabilise their condition.** This gives more time for further investigations, treatment and diagnosis.
9. **Keep calm.** Remember – it can take a few minutes for treatments to work.

Figure 2.5 Look, listen and feel

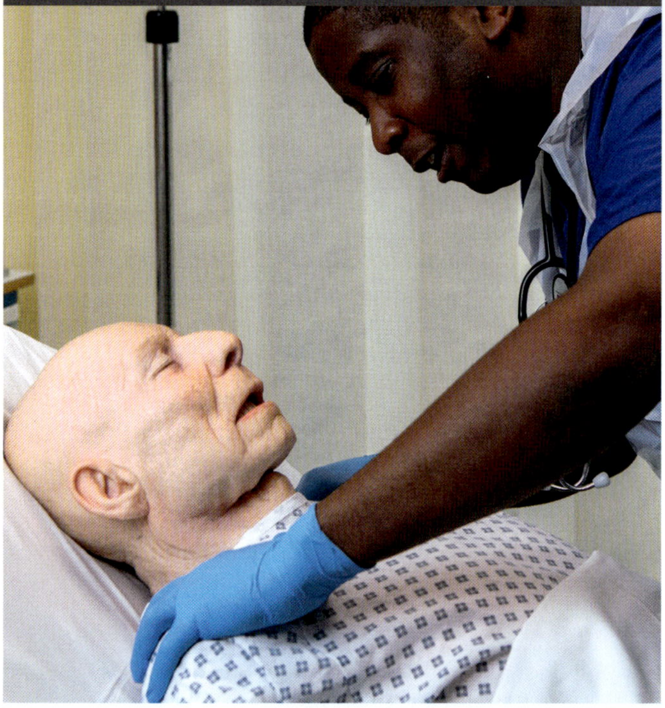

Initial approach

Look, listen and feel.

Ensure personal safety.
Wear personal protective equipment as appropriate.

Your first impression is important.
Look at the patient in general to see if they look unwell.

If they are awake, ask "How are you?"
If they appear unconscious or have collapsed, stimulate them and ask, "Are you alright?"
If they respond by talking normally, they have a patent airway, are breathing and have brain perfusion. If they speak only in short sentences, they may have breathing problems. If they do not respond, then this is concerning as they are likely to be critically ill.

If the patient is unconscious, unresponsive, and is not breathing normally (occasional gasps are not normal) **start CPR** according to the guidance in Chapter 7.
If you are confident and trained to do so, feel for a central pulse to determine if the patient has a respiratory arrest. If there are any doubts about the presence of a pulse, start CPR immediately.

This first rapid 'look, listen and feel' of the patient will often tell you a patient is critically ill and there is a need for urgent help. Ask a colleague to ensure appropriate help is coming (Figure 2.5).

A = Airway

Assess the airway and look for the signs of airway obstruction. Airway obstruction causes paradoxical chest and abdominal movements ('see-saw' respirations) and the use of the accessory muscles of respiration. Central cyanosis is a late sign of airway obstruction.

In complete airway obstruction, there are no breath sounds at the mouth or nose.

In partial obstruction, air entry is diminished and often noisy.

In the critically ill patient, depressed consciousness often leads to airway obstruction, especially if they are laying flat on their back, or if they are sitting up and their head has fallen forwards.

1. **Airway obstruction is a medical emergency and requires immediate treatment**

- In most cases, simple methods of airway clearance are all that are required (e.g. airway opening manoeuvres, suction of the airway, insertion of an oropharyngeal or nasopharyngeal airway).
- Advanced airway techniques such as insertion of a supraglottic airway or tracheal intubation may be required when these fail.

2. **Give oxygen at high-concentration**

- Give high-concentration oxygen using a mask with oxygen reservoir. Ensure that the oxygen flow is sufficient (usually 15 L min^{-1}) to prevent collapse of the oxygen reservoir bag during inspiration.
- Adjust the amount of oxygen being administered by monitoring the oxygen saturation with a pulse oximeter. Aim to maintain an oxygen saturation of 94–98%. In patients at risk of hypercapnic respiratory failure (see below), aim for an oxygen saturation of 88–92%.

B = Breathing

Diagnose and treat life-threatening conditions early (e.g. acute severe asthma, pulmonary oedema, tension pneumothorax, and massive haemothorax).

1. **Look, listen and feel for the general signs of respiratory distress.**

- Sweating, use of the accessory muscles, abdominal breathing and central cyanosis. (Central cyanosis can be identified by the mucus membranes, lips, or tongue that may appear blue or grey).
- Count the respiratory rate. The normal rate is 12–20 breaths min^{-1}. A high (> 25 min^{-1}) or increasing respiratory rate is often a marker of illness and a warning that the patient may deteriorate suddenly.
- Assess the depth of each breath, the pattern (rhythm) of respiration and whether chest expansion is equal and normal on both sides.
- Note any chest deformity (this can increase the risk of deterioration in the ability to breathe normally). Note the presence and patency of any chest drains. Remember that abdominal distension can limit diaphragmatic movement, thereby worsening respiratory distress.

2. **Record the inspired oxygen concentration (%) and the SpO_2 reading of the pulse oximeter.**

- The pulse oximeter measures blood oxygen saturation only. If the patient is receiving supplemental oxygen, the SpO_2 may be normal even with inadequate ventilation and hypercapnia (a raised level of carbon dioxide in the blood and an indicator of respiratory failure).
- Listen to the patient's breath sounds: rattling airway noises indicate the presence of airway secretions, usually because the patient cannot cough or take a deep breath. Audible stridor (an upper airway noise on inspiration) or wheeze (on expiration) suggests partial, but significant, airway obstruction.
- Percuss the chest if you are trained to do so. Hyper-resonance suggests a pneumothorax; dullness usually indicates consolidation or pleural fluid.
- Auscultate the chest with a stethoscope if you are trained to do so. Bronchial breathing indicates lung consolidation with patent airways; absent or reduced sounds suggest a pneumothorax or pleural fluid or lung consolidation.
- Check the position of the trachea in the suprasternal notch: deviation to one side indicates mediastinal shift (e.g. pneumothorax, lung fibrosis or pleural fluid). Tracheal deviation is often a late sign and difficult to identify.

Figure 2.5 Breathing

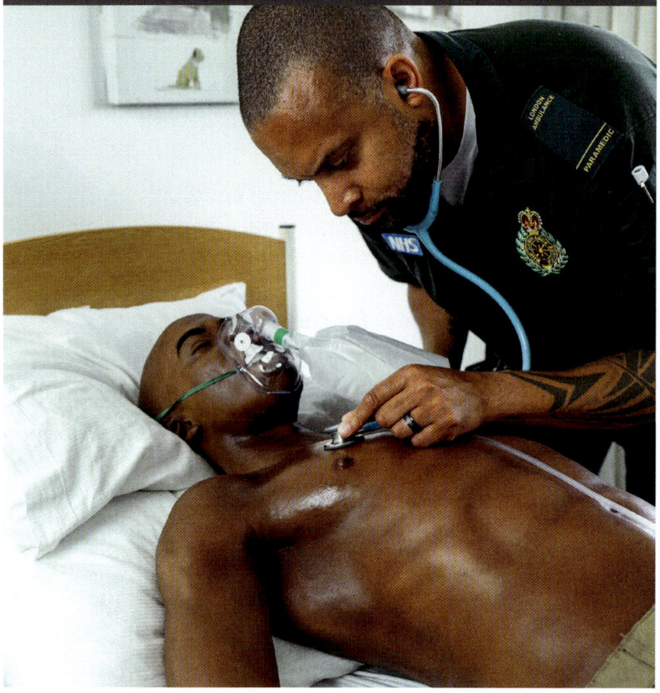

3. **Feel the chest wall to detect surgical emphysema or crepitus.**
   - This can be felt as a crackling or popping sensation under the skin and suggests a pneumothorax until proven otherwise.

4. **The treatment of respiratory disorders depends upon the cause.**
   - All critically ill patients should be given oxygen (if clinically indicated). In some patients with chronic obstructive pulmonary disease (COPD), high concentrations of oxygen can depress breathing (i.e. they are at risk of hypercapnic respiratory failure – often referred to as type II respiratory failure). Nevertheless, these patients will also sustain end-organ damage or cardiac arrest if their blood oxygen level is allowed to decrease. In this group, aim for a lower-than-normal oxygen saturation. Titrate oxygen to aim for target SpO_2 range of 88–92% in most COPD patients but evaluate the target for each patient based on their arterial blood gas measurements during previous exacerbations (if available). Some patients with chronic lung disease carry an oxygen alert card (that documents their target saturation) and their own appropriate Venturi mask.
   - If the patient's depth or rate of breathing is inadequate or absent, use two-person bag-mask or pocket mask ventilation to improve oxygenation and ventilation, whilst calling immediately for expert help. In cooperative patients who do not have an airway obstruction, consider the use of non-invasive ventilation (NIV). In patients with an acute exacerbation of COPD, the use of NIV is often helpful and prevents the need for tracheal intubation and invasive ventilation.

C = Circulation

In almost all medical and surgical emergencies, consider hypovolaemia to be the likeliest cause of shock, unless proven otherwise. Unless there are obvious signs of a cardiac cause (e.g. chest pain, heart failure), give intravenous fluid to a patient with cool peripheries and a fast heart rate.

In surgical patients, rapidly exclude bleeding (overt or hidden). Remember that breathing problems, such as a tension pneumothorax, can also compromise a patient's circulatory state. This should have been treated earlier in the assessment.

1. **Look at the colour of the hands and fingers in accordance with the patient's skin tone:** are they blue or grey, are they mottled?

2. **Hold the patient's hand:** is it cool or warm?

3. **Measure the capillary refill time (CRT).**
   - Apply pressure for 5 seconds centrally or on a fingertip held at heart level (or just above) with enough pressure to cause blanching. Time how long it takes for the area to return to the colour of the surrounding skin after releasing the pressure. In individuals with black and brown skin, it may be more appropriate to turn the hand over and perform the CRT on the palmer-side of the finger where it may be easier to observe objectively.
   - The normal value for CRT is usually less than 2 s. A prolonged CRT suggests poor peripheral perfusion. Other factors (e.g. cold surroundings, poor lighting, advanced age) can prolong CRT.

4. **Count the patient's pulse rate and feel the peripheral and central (carotid) pulses.**
   - Assess for presence, rate, quality, regularity and equality. Barely palpable central pulses suggest a poor cardiac output, whilst a bounding pulse can indicate sepsis.
   - Measure the patient's blood pressure. Even in shock, the blood pressure may be normal, because compensatory mechanisms increase peripheral resistance in response to reduced cardiac output. A low diastolic blood pressure suggests arterial vasodilation (as in anaphylaxis or sepsis). A narrowed pulse pressure (difference between systolic and diastolic pressures; normally 35–45 mmHg) suggests arterial vasoconstriction (cardiogenic shock or hypovolaemia).
   - Auscultate the heart with a stethoscope if you are trained to do so. Is there a murmur or pericardial rub? Are the heart sounds difficult to hear? Does the audible heart rate correspond to the pulse rate?

- Look for other signs of a poor cardiac output, such as reduced conscious level and, if the patient has a urinary catheter, oliguria (urine volume less than 0.5 mL kg^{-1} h^{-1}).
- Look thoroughly for external bleeding from wounds or drains or evidence of concealed bleeding (e.g. thoracic, intraperitoneal, retroperitoneal or into the gut). Intrathoracic, intra-abdominal or pelvic blood loss can be significant, even if drains are empty.

5. **The treatment of cardiovascular collapse depends on the cause,** but should be directed at fluid replacement, bleeding control and restoration of tissue perfusion.

- Look for the signs which are immediately life-threatening (e.g. cardiac tamponade, massive or continuing bleeding, sepsis) and treat them urgently.

6. **If trained to do so, insert one or more large (14 or 16 G) intravenous cannulae.**

- Use short, wide-bore cannulae, because they enable the highest flow.

7. **Take blood from a cannula** for routine haematological, biochemical, coagulation, microbiological investigations, and cross-matching, before infusing intravenous fluid.

- Measuring a temperature before will help determine if blood cultures are also indicated.
- Give a rapid bolus of 500 mL of crystalloid solution (e.g. Hartmann's solution or 0.9% sodium chloride) over less than 15 minutes. Use smaller volumes (e.g. 250 mL) for patients with known cardiac failure or trauma and monitor closely (listen to the chest for crackles after each bolus if trained to do so).
- Reassess the heart rate and BP regularly (every 5 minutes), aiming for the patient's normal BP or, if this is unknown, a target > 100 mmHg systolic.
- If the patient does not improve, repeat the fluid challenge. Seek expert help if there is a lack of response to repeated fluid boluses. Lack of response can indicate bleeding.
- If signs and symptoms of cardiac failure (dyspnoea, increased heart rate, raised jugular venous pressure (JVP), a third heart sound and pulmonary crackles on auscultation) occur, decrease the fluid infusion rate or stop the fluids altogether. Ask for expert help as other treatments that improve tissue perfusion (e.g. inotropes or vasopressors) may be needed.
- If the patient has chest pain and a suspected ACS, record a 12-lead ECG early, and treat initially with aspirin, nitroglycerine, oxygen (if saturations are below the target range), and morphine.

D = Disability

Common causes of unconsciousness include profound hypoxia, hypercapnia, cerebral hypoperfusion due to a low blood pressure, sedatives or analgesic drugs.

1. **Review and treat the ABCs:** exclude or treat hypoxia and hypotension.

2. **Check the patient's drug chart for reversible drug-induced causes of depressed consciousness.** Give an antagonist where appropriate (e.g. naloxone for opioid toxicity).

3. **Examine the pupils** (size, equality and reaction to light).

4. **Make a rapid initial assessment of the patient's conscious level using the ACVPU method:**
   A = **A**lert
   C = new **C**onfusion
   V = responds to **V**ocal stimulus
   P = responds to **P**ainful stimulus or
   U = **U**nresponsive to all stimulus.

   Alternatively, use the Glasgow Coma Scale score. A painful stimulus can be given by squeezing the trapezius muscle.

5. **Measure the blood glucose** to exclude hypoglycaemia using a rapid finger-prick bedside testing method.

- In the sickest patients, blood should be taken from a vein or artery as finger prick samples may not be as reliable for blood glucose measurements.
- Follow local protocols for management of hypoglycaemia. For example, if the blood sugar is below 4.0 mmol L^{-1} in an unconscious patient, give an initial dose of 50 mL of 10% glucose solution intravenously. If necessary, give further doses of intravenous 10% glucose every minute until the patient has fully regained consciousness, or a total of 250 mL of 10% glucose has been given. Repeat blood glucose measurements to monitor the effects of treatment. If there is no improvement, consider further doses of 10% glucose. Specific national guidance exists for the management of hypoglycaemia in adults with diabetes mellitus.

6. **Consider placing unconscious patients in the lateral position** if their airway is not protected.

E = Exposure

1. **Examine for rashes, bruising, bleeding and any other noted abnormalities.**

- Be aware that rashes can present differently across different skin tones. Urticaria may be visible as a red or pink rash but this may be less apparent in some skin tones, but can be detected as raised areas of skin.
- If not already done, record the patient's temperature.

Figure 2.6 Exposure

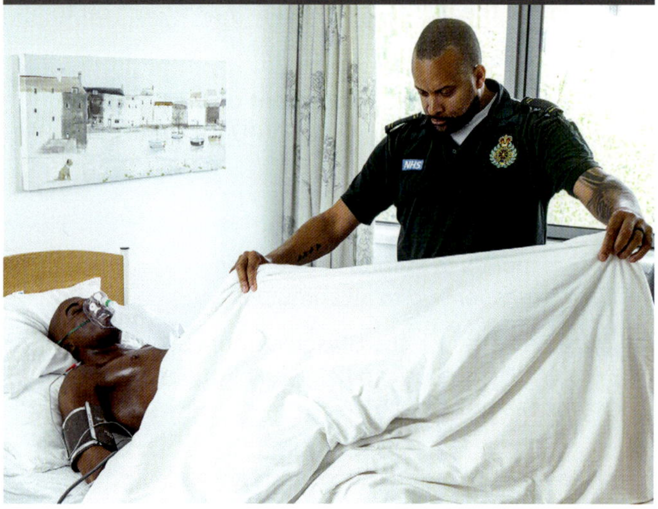

Additional information

1. **Take a full clinical history** from the patient, any relatives or friends, and other staff.
2. **Review the patient's notes and charts:**
   - Review trended values of vital signs, in addition to current observations.
   - Check that important routine medications are prescribed and being given.
   - Review the results of laboratory or radiological investigations.
3. **Make complete entries in the patient's notes** of your findings, assessment and treatment. Record the patient's response to therapy. Where necessary, handover the patient to your colleagues using **SBARD** or **RSVP** (Table 4.1).
4. **Consider which level of care is required** by the patient (e.g. emergency department, ward, HDU, ICU) and what definitive treatment is appropriate for the patient's underlying condition.
5. **Keep the patient and relatives informed** of what is happening.

02 SUMMARY LEARNING

Most patients who have an in-hospital cardiac arrest have warning signs and symptoms before the arrest.

Early recognition and treatment of the deteriorating patient will prevent some cardiac arrests.

Use strategies such as National Early Warning Score 2 (NEWS2) to identify patients at risk of deterioration and cardiac arrest.

Airway, breathing and circulation problems can cause cardiac arrest.

Use the ABCDE assessment to assess and treat critically ill patients.

TEST YOURSELF QUESTIONS

1. What are 3 potential causes of airway obstruction?
2. What are the signs and symptoms of breathing problems?
3. How do you measure a capillary refill time?
4. When palpating a pulse during a circulatory assessment, besides rate, what other information can be obtained?

Further reading

Drennan IR, Greif R, Bray JE, et al., on behalf of the ILCOR Advanced Life Support Task Force. 2025 International Consensus on Cardiopulmonary Resuscitation and Emergency Cardiovascular Care Science With Treatment Recommendations. Advanced Life Support. ILCOR, 2025. In print.

Intensive Care National Audit & Research Centre (2024) National Cardiac Arrest Audit: Summary Statistics 2022–23. London: ICNARC. Available at: https://www.icnarc.org/wp-content/uploads/2024/05/NCAA-Summary-Statistics-2022-23.pdf.pdf (Accessed: 10 July 2025).

National Early Warning Score (NEWS) 2: Standardising the assessment of acute-illness severity in the NHS. Updated report of a working party. Royal College of Physicians, London, 2017.

NICE clinical guideline 50 Acutely ill patients in-hospital: recognition of and response to acute illness in adults in hospital. London: National Institute for Health and Clinical Excellence; 2007. https://www.nice.org.uk/guidance/cg50

National Institute for Health and Care Excellence. NICE Guideline 185. Acute Coronary Syndromes. 2020. https://www.nice.org.uk/guidance/ng185

Robinson EJ, Smith GB, Power GS et al Risk-adjusted survival for adults following in-hospital cardiac arrest by day of week and time of day: observational cohort study, BMJ Qual Saf 2016;25:832– 841.

National Institute for Health and Care Excellence. NICE Guideline 185. Acute Coronary Syndromes. 2020. https://www.nice.org.uk/guidance/ng185Smith GB. In-hospital cardiac arrest: Is it time for an in-hospital 'chain of prevention'? Resuscitation 2010:81:1209-11.

NHS England (n.d.) Martha's Rule. NHS England. Available at: HYPERLINK "https://www.england.nhs.uk/patient-safety/marthas-rule/?utm_source=chatgpt.com"https://www.england.nhs.uk/patient-safety/marthas-rule/

Soar J, Berg K, Andersen L, et al. Adult Advanced Life Support: 2020 International Consensus on Cardiopulmonary Resuscitation and Emergency Cardiovascular Care Science with Treatment Recommendations. Resuscitation 2020;156: PA80-A119.

Smyth M, van Goor S, Giuseppe Ristagno, Malta Hansen C. et al. European Resuscitation Council 2025: Basic Life Support. Resuscitation. 2025. In print.

Soar J, Böttiger B, Carli P, et al. European Resuscitation Council Guidelines 2025: Advanced Life Support. Resuscitation. 2025. In print.

The Hospital Management of Hypoglycaemia in Adults with Diabetes Mellitus. Joint British Diabetes Societies. Revised 2013.

Vaillancourt C, Olasveengen TM, Bray JE, et al., on behalf of the ILCOR Basic Life Support Task Force. 2025 International Consensus on Cardiopulmonary Resuscitation and Emergency Cardiovascular Care Science With Treatment Recommendations. Basic Life Support. ILCOR, 2025. In print.

My key take-home messages from this chapter are:

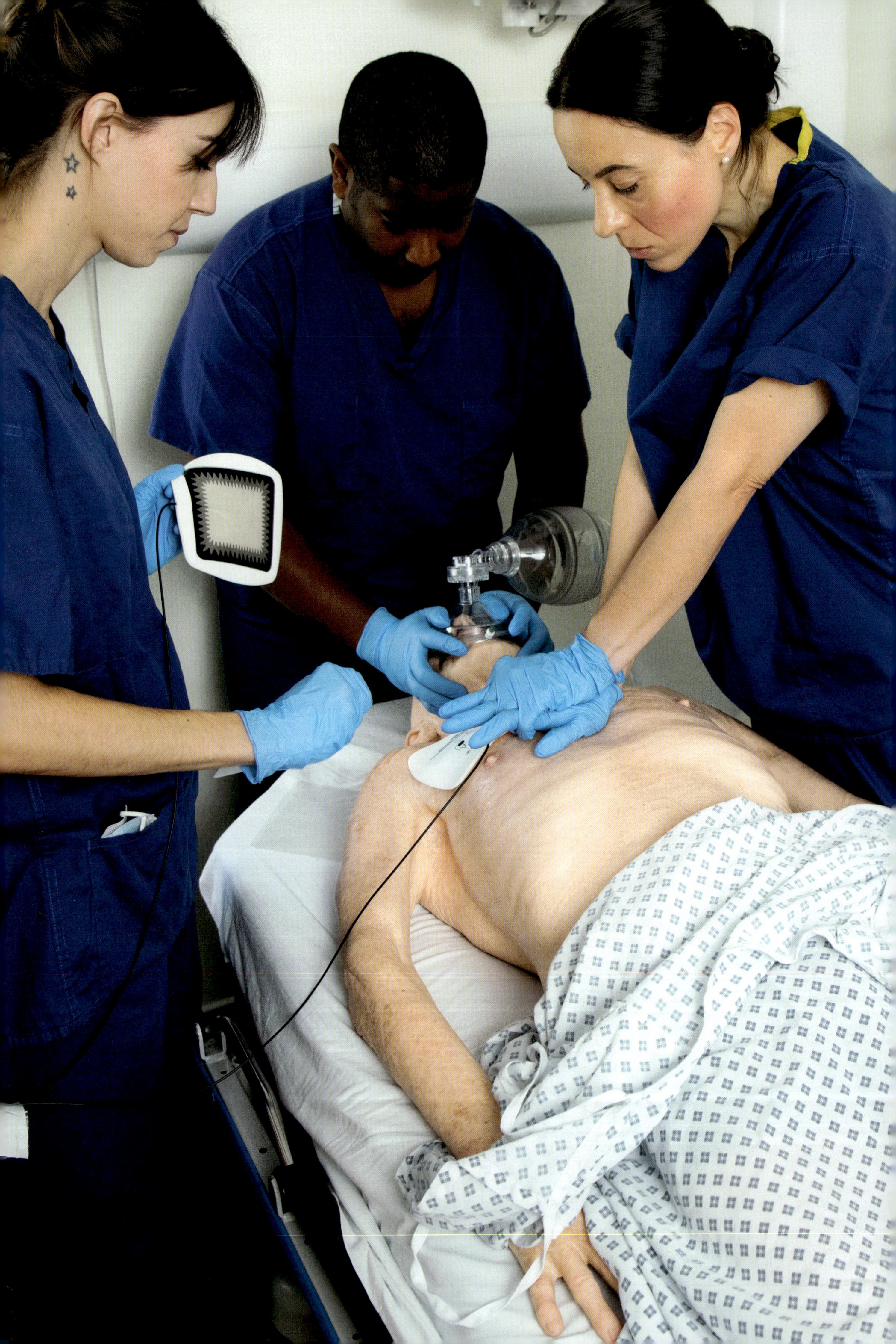

03 Immediate resuscitation

In this chapter

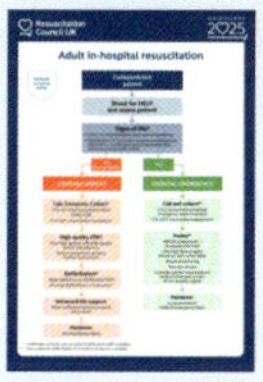

The adult in-hospital resuscitation algorithm

The Chain of Survival

Features specific to resuscitation by trained responders

Sequence for the collapsed patient in a healthcare setting

The mechanism of defibrillation and factors affecting defibrillation success

The sequence for safe use of automated external defibrillators (AED) and/or manual defibrillators

The learning outcomes will enable you to:

Start immediate resuscitation

Give high-quality cardiopulmonary resuscitation (CPR) with minimal interruption

Understand how to safely deliver a shock with an AED and/or manual defibrillator

Understand the importance of minimising pauses in chest compressions during CPR/ defibrillation

Continue resuscitation until more experienced help arrives

This chapter is intended for healthcare professionals who are the first to respond to a cardiac arrest. It is applicable to healthcare professionals working in hospitals, as well as those working in other clinical settings, such as community hospitals, mental health hospitals, primary care and for out-of-hospital providers such as ambulance service clinicians.

The Chain of Survival

The Chain of Survival (Figure 3.1) describes the interventions that contribute to patient survival. The strength of the whole chain is dependent on the strength of each of the four links. They are:

1. **Early recognition and call for help – to prevent cardiac arrest**
2. **Early CPR and defibrillation to preserve brain and restart the heart**
3. **Advance and post-resuscitation care to optimise brain and heart function**
4. **Survival and recovery to restore quality of life.**

The public expects that all clinical staff know how to perform cardiopulmonary resuscitation (CPR).

For every cardiac arrest, ensure that:

- **cardiac arrest is recognised immediately**
- **help is summoned using a standard telephone number in acute hospitals (2222 is recommended in the UK). In community hospitals, help is usually summoned dialling 999 for an ambulance**
- **CPR is started immediately and, if indicated, defibrillation is attempted as soon as possible (within 3 minutes).**

Figure 3.1 The Chain of Survival

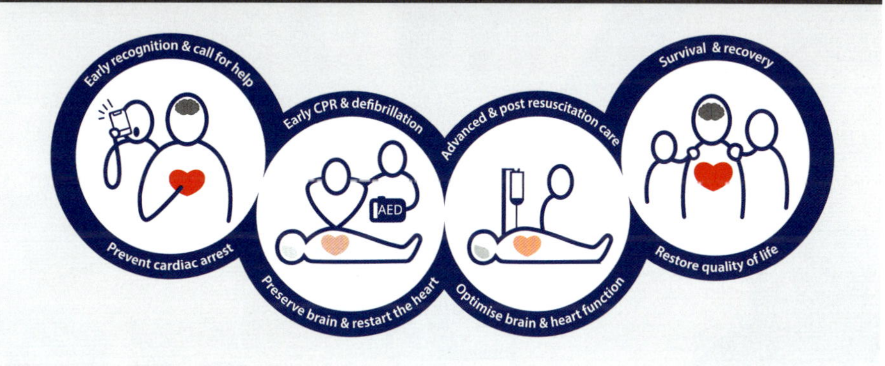

Following the onset of ventricular fibrillation or pulseless ventricular tachycardia (VF/pVT), cardiac output ceases, and cerebral hypoxic injury starts within 3 minutes.

For complete neurological recovery, early successful defibrillation with return of spontaneous circulation (ROSC) is essential.

Defibrillation is a key link in the Chain of Survival and is one of the few interventions with high quality evidence to demonstrate that it is independently associated with significantly improved outcomes from VF/pVT cardiac arrests. The shorter the interval between the onset of VF/pVT and delivery of the shock, the greater the chance of successful defibrillation and survival.

Defibrillators with automated rhythm recognition (automated external defibrillators (AEDs)) are reliable, computerised devices designed to use voice and visual prompts to guide lay rescuers and healthcare professionals to attempt defibrillation safely in cardiac arrest patients (Figure 3.2). Sufficient staff should be trained to enable the first shock to be delivered within 3 minutes of collapse anywhere in a healthcare setting.

Why is in-hospital resuscitation different?

The exact sequence of actions after cardiac arrest depends on several factors, and this will vary depending on the setting, particularly if in an acute hospital compared to a community healthcare setting or out of hospital setting.

Other factors that will influence the response are:

- location (clinical/non-clinical area, monitored/unmonitored area)
- skills of the first responders
- number of responders
- equipment available
- rapid response system to cardiac arrest and medical emergencies (e.g. medical emergency team (MET), resuscitation team).

Location of cardiac arrest

Patients who have a witnessed or monitored cardiac arrest in an acute care area are usually diagnosed and treated quickly. Ideally, all patients who are at high risk of cardiac arrest should be cared for in a monitored area where staff and facilities for immediate resuscitation are available. Patients, visitors or staff may also have a cardiac arrest in non-clinical areas of hospitals (e.g. car parks, corridors), and it may be necessary to move the patient to enable continued resuscitation.

Figure 3.2 Use of AED during immediate resuscitation

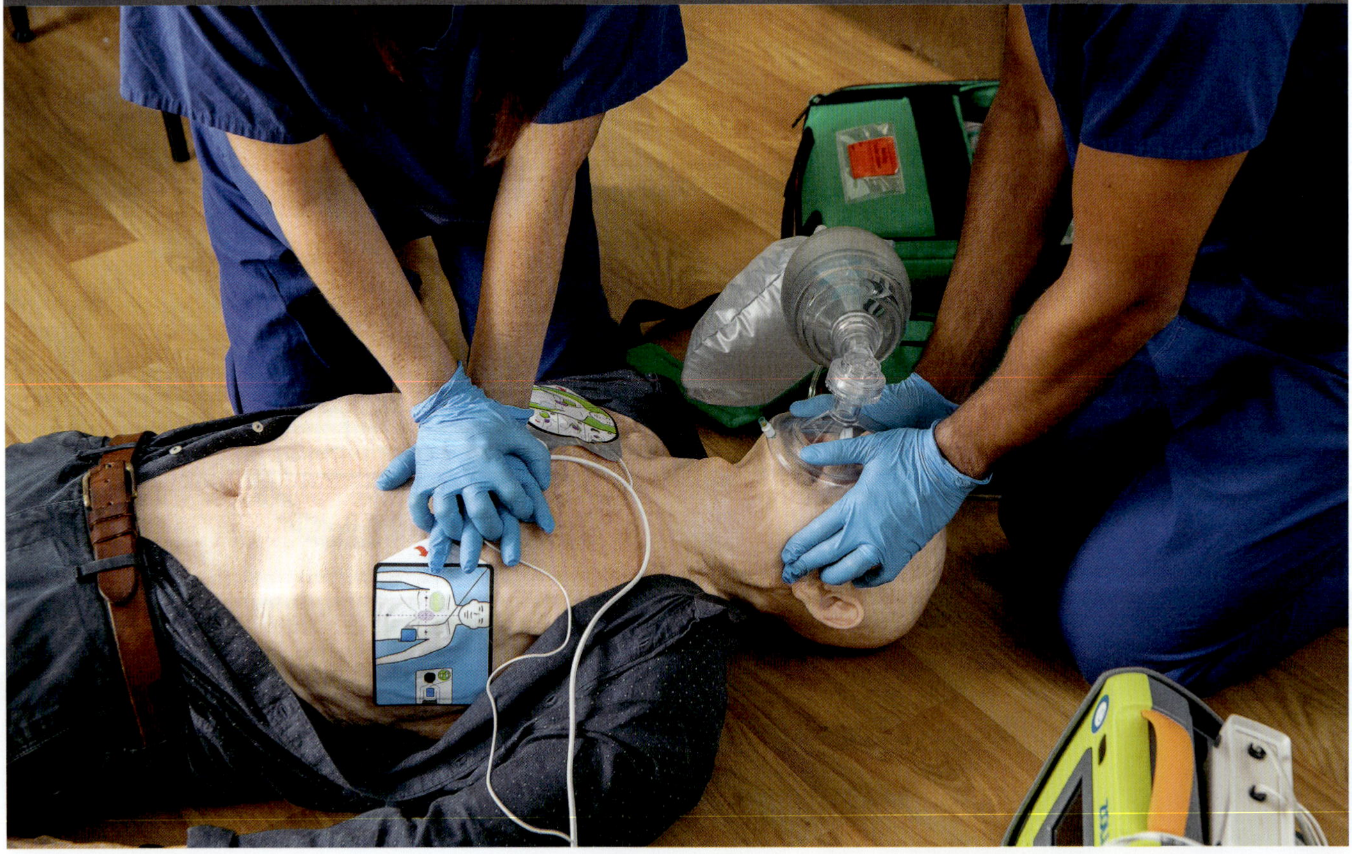

Skills of first responders

Those with a responsibility to respond should be able to recognise cardiac arrest, call for help and start chest compressions. They should do what they have been trained to do. For example, those working in critical care and emergency medicine may have more advanced resuscitation skills and greater experience in resuscitation than those who rarely use resuscitation skills. Use the skills you are trained to do. Individuals should only use a manual defibrillator if they are trained, competent, and confident in its use. Otherwise, an AED or a manual defibrillator in AED mode must be used.

Number of responders

Always ensure that help is on the way. Usually, colleagues are nearby and several actions can be undertaken simultaneously.

Equipment available

Responders should have immediate access to resuscitation equipment and medications. Ideally, the equipment used for cardiopulmonary resuscitation (including defibrillators) and the layout of equipment and medications should be standardised throughout the hospital. You should be familiar with the resuscitation equipment used in your clinical area. This may not be practical in some clinical settings or for out-of-hospital teams who may be unaware they will later form part of a resuscitation team together.

Out-of-hospital providers should use standardised response bags with easily accessible resuscitation equipment including a defibrillator that can be carried to any emergency where there is potential for a cardiac arrest.

Serious patient safety incidents associated with CPR and patient deterioration are commonly associated with equipment problems during resuscitation (e.g. portable suction not working, defibrillator pads missing). Specially designed trolleys or sealed tray systems can enhance the speed of equipment access and reduce the risk of adverse incidents. Resuscitation equipment or response bags with dedicated tagged resuscitation pouches must be checked regularly to ensure they are ready for use.

AEDs can be used in both clinical and non-clinical areas where staff lack rhythm recognition skills or rarely need to use a defibrillator. This type of defibrillator is often found in community settings and is usually in wall-mounted cabinets that sometimes require a key code from the ambulance service. The use of AEDs can deliver a much-needed shock during the precious minutes before the arrival of the resuscitation team or ambulance service responders. Some healthcare providers may have mechanical CPR devices; follow local policies and the manufacturer's instructions for use and training.

Figure 3.3 The resuscitation team

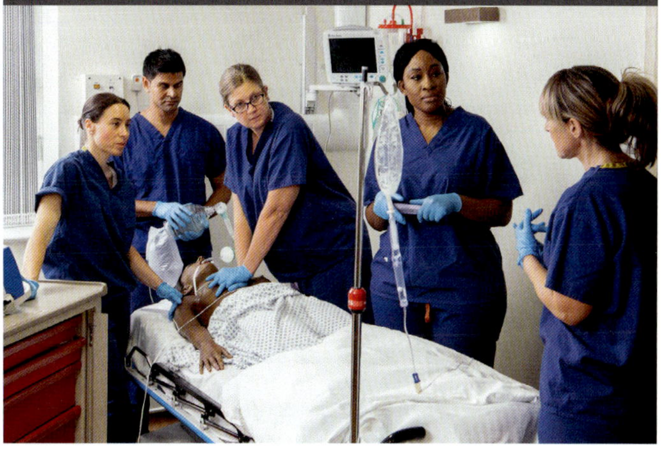

Waveform capnography is a monitor that is routinely used during anaesthesia and for critically ill patients requiring mechanical ventilation. It must be used to confirm correct tracheal tube placement during resuscitation and can also help guide resuscitation interventions (Chapter 7). It can also be used after supraglottic insertion.

Waveform capnography monitoring is available on newer defibrillators, as part of portable monitors or as a hand-held device.

After successful resuscitation, patients often need to be transferred to other clinical areas (e.g. intensive care unit) or other hospitals. Ensure transfer equipment and drugs are available to enable this to be done safely. In community settings, patients will be transferred to hospital by the ambulance service, which will provide their own equipment.

At the end of every resuscitation attempt, ensure that equipment and drugs are replaced immediately and are readily available for use the next time they are needed.

Resuscitation team

The resuscitation team (Figure 3.3) can be a traditional cardiac arrest team, which is only called when a cardiac arrest is recognised. In some hospitals, a rapid response team (e.g. medical emergency team (MET)) is called if a patient is deteriorating before cardiac arrest occurs.

Resuscitation team members should ideally meet at the beginning of each shift for introductions and allocation of specific roles. This may not be practical in some clinical settings or for out-of-hospital teams who may be unaware they will later form part of a resuscitation team together. In the out of hospital setting, the resuscitation team will comprise of those responders who have been assigned to the incident, and it may evolve over time as more resources arrive. Knowing each other's names, skills, and experience, and discussing how the team will work together during a resuscitation, will improve teamwork during resuscitation attempts. Team members should debrief after each event to enable open discussion of performance and concerns. This has most benefit when discussions are based on data collected during the event (Chapter 4).

Figure 3.4 Manual defibrillator

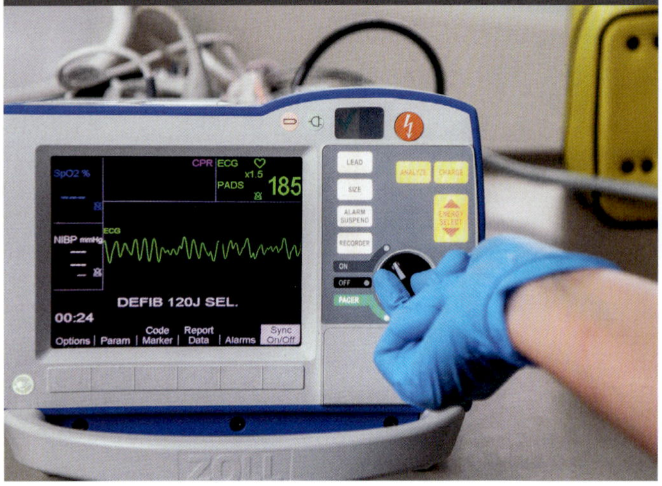

Figure 3.5a Standard electrode position

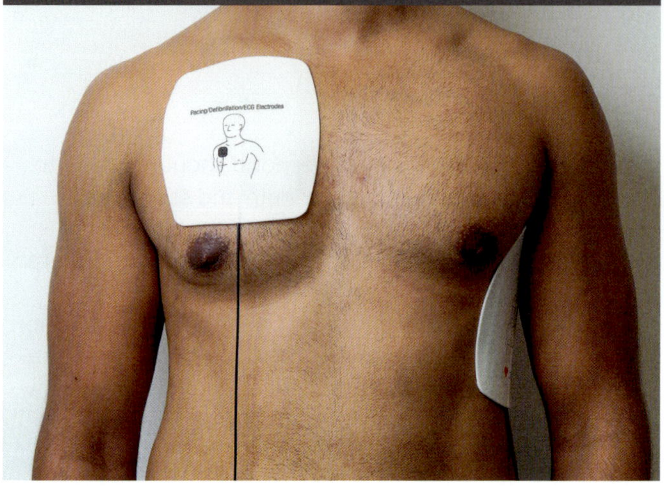

Principles of safe and effective defibrillation

Defibrillation is the passage of an electrical current across the myocardium to depolarise a critical mass of heart muscle simultaneously, enabling the natural 'pacemaker' tissue to resume control.

Factors affecting defibrillation success

Defibrillation success depends on sufficient current being delivered to the myocardium. Factors affecting defibrillation success include:

- transthoracic impedance
- electrode position
- the shock energy, and
- the shock sequence.

Transthoracic impedance

Transthoracic impedance is the resistance of the thorax to electric current flow. Some defibrillators measure the transthoracic impedance through their defibrillator pads and adjust their output accordingly, which is known as impedance compensation. To minimise the impedance:

- Ensure good contact between self-adhesive pads and the patient's skin. Use the self-adhesive pads recommended by the manufacturer for the specific defibrillator.
- If the patient has a very hairy chest, and a razor is immediately available, use it to shave the area where the electrodes are placed. Ensure chest compressions continue while shaving the chest. However, defibrillation should not be delayed if a razor is not to hand immediately.
- Remove drug-eluting patches or transdermal patches if in the area where the self-adhesive pads would be applied. If this is likely to delay defibrillation, place the pads in an alternative position that avoids the patch.

Electrode position

The electrodes (also known as defibrillator pads or self-adhesive pads) are positioned to achieve the greatest current flow through the myocardium. Pads placed in the correct position greatly increase the chance of a shock being successful. The standard positions are one electrode to the right of the upper sternum, below the clavicle; the lateral (apical) pad is positioned directly below the armpit in the mid-axillary line, clear of breast tissue (ensure it is sufficiently lateral (Figure 3.5 a,b)).

Other acceptable positions include:

- One electrode anteriorly, over the left precordium, and the other electrode on the back behind the heart, just inferior to the left scapula (antero-posterior).
- One electrode is placed in the standard apical position, and the other electrode is on the back, over the right scapula (postero-lateral).
- The lateral chest walls, one on the right and the other on the left side (bi-axillary) (Figure 3.6).

There should only be a brief pause in compressions to apply a CPR feedback device in the correct position.

Shock sequence

For all cardiac arrests, start CPR immediately. Use the defibrillator to assess the rhythm as soon as it arrives. Although defibrillation is key to the management of patients in VF/pVT, continuous, uninterrupted chest compressions are also required to optimise the chances of successful resuscitation. Even short interruptions in chest compressions (e.g. to deliver rescue breaths or perform rhythm analysis) reduce the chances of successful defibrillation. The aim is to ensure that chest compressions are performed continuously throughout the resuscitation attempt, pausing briefly only to enable specific interventions.

Another factor critical to determining the success of defibrillation is the duration of the pre-shock pause, the interval between stopping chest compressions and delivering the shock. Every 5-second increase in the pre-shock pause almost halves the chance of successful defibrillation.

Figure 3.5b Lateral pad position

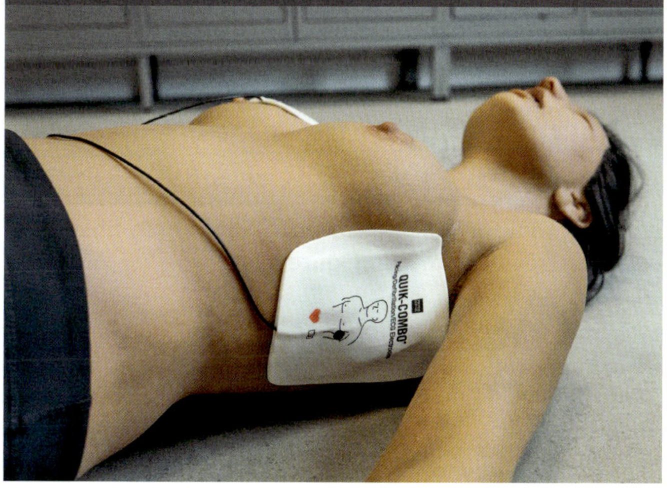

Consequently, defibrillation must always be performed quickly and efficiently to maximise the chances of successful resuscitation. If there is any delay in obtaining a defibrillator, continue high-quality chest compressions and ventilation while the defibrillator pads are being applied.

Defibrillator safety

Do not deliver a shock if anybody is touching the patient. Do not hold intravenous infusion equipment or the patient's trolley/bed during the delivery of shock. The operator must ensure that everyone is clear of the patient before delivering a shock. Wipe any water or fluids from the patient's chest before attempting defibrillation. The gloves routinely available in clinical settings do not provide sufficient protection from the electric current; therefore, a shock must only be delivered when everyone is clear of the patient.

Safe use of oxygen during defibrillation

Sparks in an oxygen-enriched atmosphere can cause fire and burns to the patient. Self-adhesive pads are far less likely to cause sparks than manual paddles. The following precautions reduce the risk of fire:

- Remove any oxygen mask or nasal cannulae and place them at least one metre away from the patient's chest.
- Leave the self-inflating bag connected to the tracheal tube or well-fitted supraglottic airway as no increase in oxygen concentration occurs in the zone of defibrillation, even with an oxygen flow of 15 L min^{-1}. Alternatively, disconnect the ventilation bag from the tracheal tube or supraglottic airway and remove it at least one metre from the patient's chest during defibrillation.
- If the patient is connected to a ventilator, for example, in the operating room or critical care unit, leave the ventilator tubing (breathing circuit) connected to the tracheal tube unless chest compressions prevent the ventilator from delivering adequate tidal volumes. In this case, the ventilator is usually substituted by a self-inflating bag, which can be left connected or detached and removed to a distance of at least one metre. If the ventilator tubing is disconnected, ensure it is kept at least one metre from the patient, or better still, switch the ventilator off. Modern ventilators generate massive oxygen flows when disconnected.

Figure 3.6 Alternative electrode position – bi-axillary

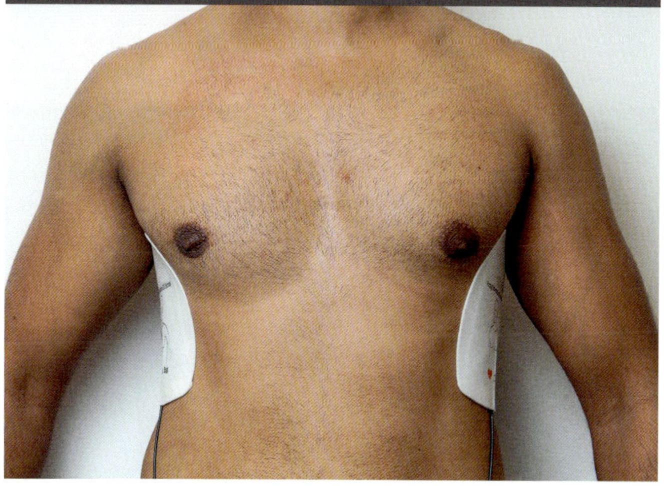

Automated rhythm analysis

It is almost impossible to shock inappropriately with an AED. Movement is usually sensed, so movement artefact is unlikely to be interpreted as a shockable rhythm.

Implanted electronic devices

When a patient needs external defibrillation, effective measures to try to restore life take priority over concerns about any implanted device such as a pacemaker, implantable cardioverter-defibrillator (ICD), implantable event recorder or neurostimulator. Current resuscitation guidelines are followed, but awareness of the presence of an implanted device allows some additional measures to optimise outcome:

- To minimise the risk of damage to the device, place the defibrillator electrodes away from the pacemaker or ICD generator (at least 8 cm) without compromising effective defibrillation. If necessary, place the pads in the antero-posterior, postero-lateral or bi-axillary position as described above.
- An ICD gives no warning when it delivers a shock. In an emergency, a ring magnet can be placed over the ICD to deactivate the defibrillation function if necessary. Deactivation of an ICD in this manner does not disable the device's ability to act as a pacemaker if it has that capability.
- During a shockable rhythm, external defibrillation should be attempted in the usual way if the ICD has not delivered a shock, or if its shocks have failed to terminate the arrhythmia.
- In refractory VF/pVT, consider changing the pad position by applying new pads in the AP position.

Figure 3.7 Head tilt and chin lift

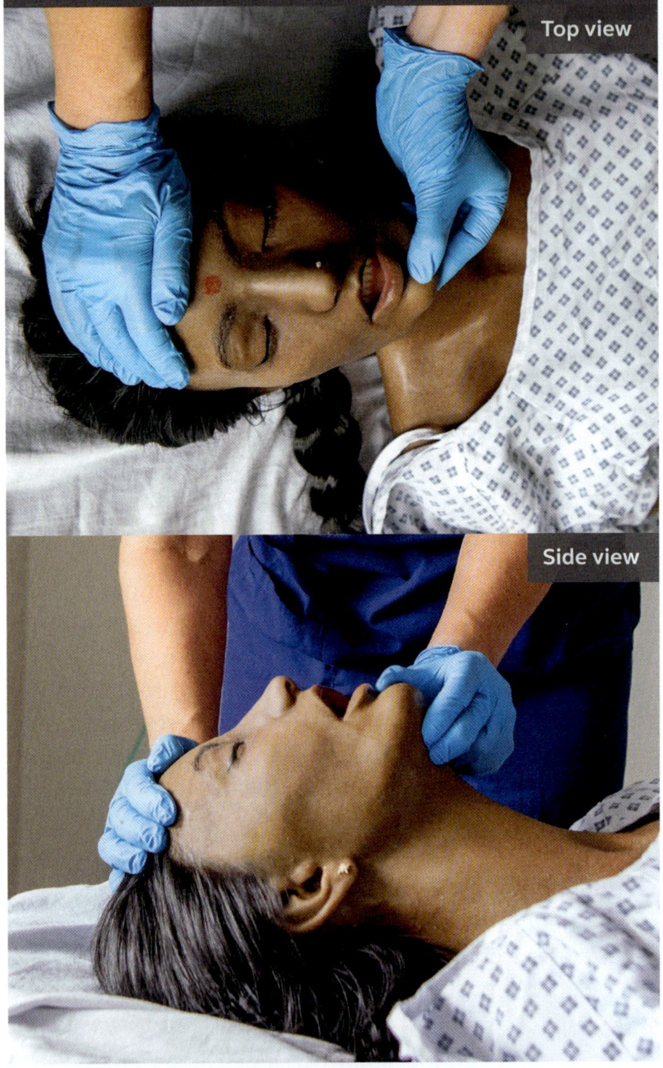

Figure 3.8 Check the patient for a response – shake and shout "are you alright?"

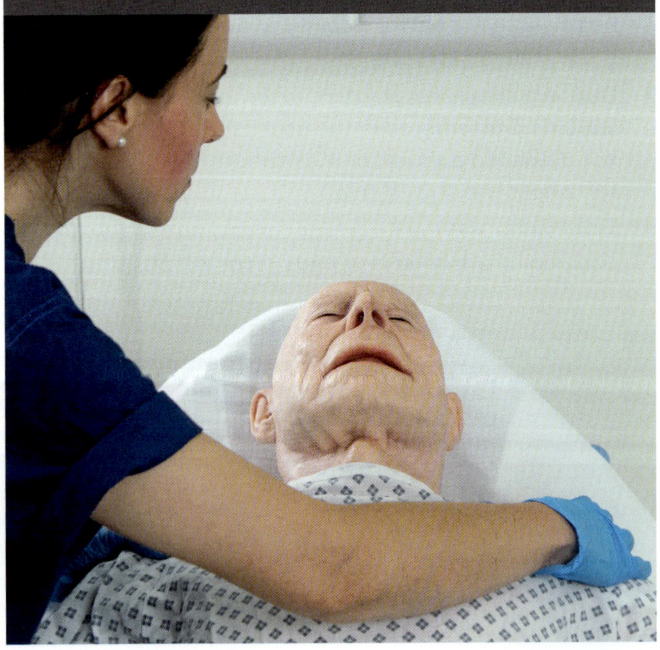

Adult in-hospital resuscitation – the sequence for a collapsed patient

An algorithm for the initial management of in-hospital cardiac arrest is shown in Figure 3.9.

1. Ensure personal safety

There are very few reports of harm to rescuers during resuscitation. Your own safety and that of resuscitation team members is the first priority.

- Check that the patient's surroundings are safe.
- Put on personal protective equipment (PPE) (e.g. gloves, eye protection, face masks, aprons, gowns) as appropriate. Follow national and local infection control measures and PPE guidelines from your employer.
- Be careful with sharps; a sharps box must be available.
- Use safe handling techniques for moving individuals during resuscitation.
- Avoid contact with corrosive chemicals or substances such as organophosphates that are easily absorbed through the skin or respiratory tract. Care should be taken when resuscitating patients who have had radioactive treatment.
- Defibrillator safety as discussed above.

2. Check the patient for a response

If you see a patient collapse or find a patient unconscious:

- First shout for help.
- Then assess if they are responsive by gently stimulating them and ask loudly **"Are you all right?"** (Figure 3.8).

- If other members of staff are nearby, it will be possible to undertake actions simultaneously.

3A. If they DO respond

Urgent clinical assessment is required.

- Call for help in accordance with local procedure. This may include calling a resuscitation team (e.g. MET in a hospital) or 999 in community settings. For clinicians working in an out-of-hospital setting, request additional resources. While waiting for the team, assess the patient using the ABCDE assessment (Chapter 2).

A B C D E

Adult in-hospital resuscitation

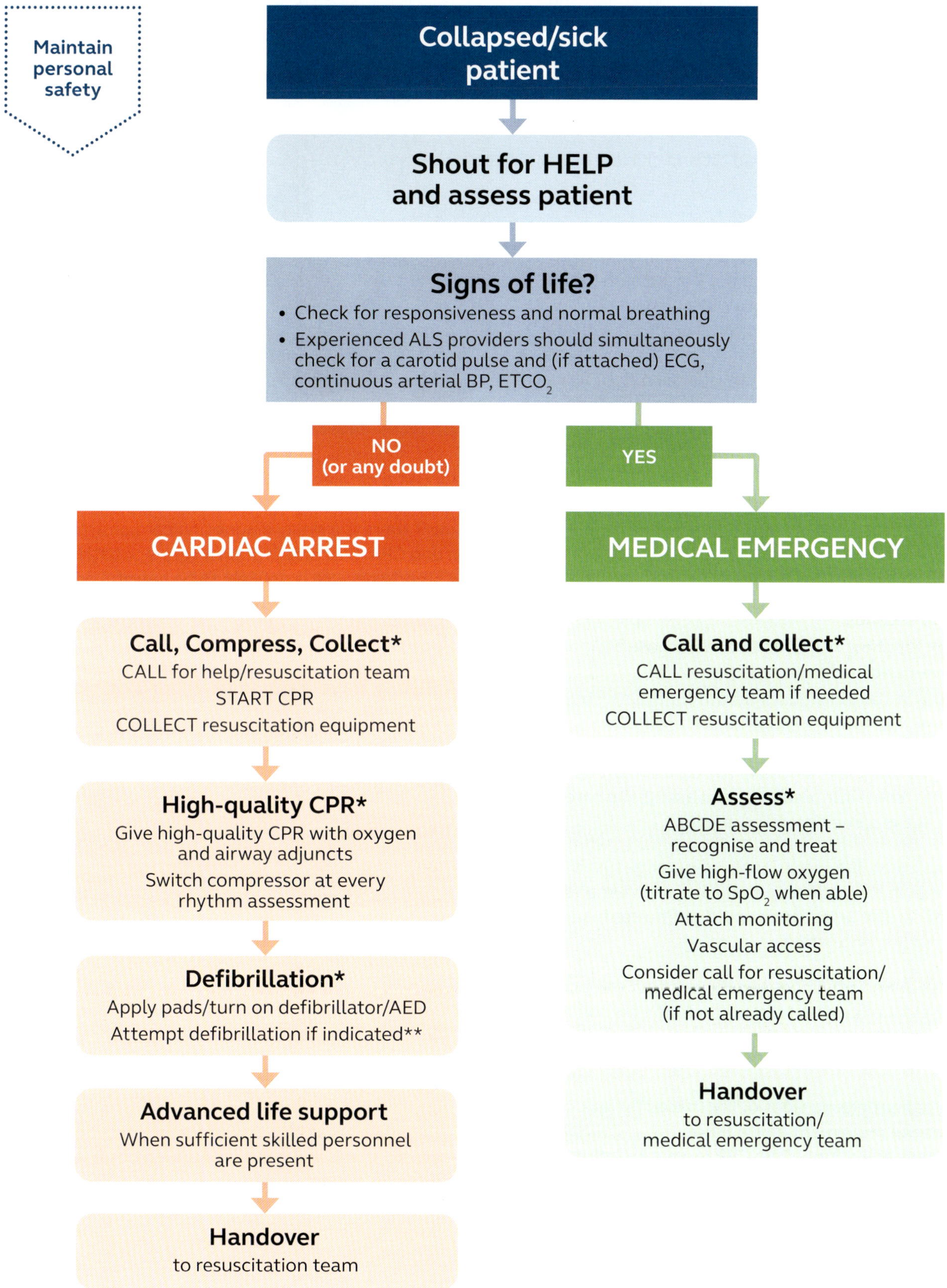

* Undertake actions concurrently if sufficient staff available
** Use a manual defibrillator if trained and device available

Figure 3.4 Adult in-hospital resuscitation algorithm

3B. If they DO NOT respond

- The exact sequence will depend on your training and experience in the assessment of breathing and circulation in sick patients.
- Shout/call for help (if not done already).
- Turn the patient onto their back.
- Open the airway using a head tilt and chin lift (Figure 3.7).
- If there is a risk of cervical spine injury, use a jaw thrust or chin lift in combination with manual in-line stabilisation of the head and neck by an assistant if available. If life-threatening airway obstruction persists despite effective application of a jaw thrust or chin lift, add a head tilt a small amount at a time until the airway is open. Establishing a patent airway, oxygenation, and ventilation must take priority over concerns about a cervical spine injury.
- Take up to 10 seconds at most to determine if the patient is in cardiac arrest.
- Keeping the airway open, look, listen and leel (Figure 3.10) to determine if the person is breathing normally. This is a rapid check and should take less than 10 seconds:
  - Look for chest rise and fall and purposeful movement.
  - Listen at the individual's mouth for breath sounds.
  - Feel for air on your cheek.
- If trained and experienced in the assessment of sick patients, check for breathing and assess the carotid pulse at the same time (Figure 3.11).
- Agonal breathing (occasional, irregular gasps) is common in the early stages of cardiac arrest and is a sign of cardiac arrest and should not be confused as a sign of life/circulation.
- A short period of seizure-like movements can occur at the start of cardiac arrest. Assess the person after the seizure has stopped; if unresponsive and not breathing normally, start CPR.
- If the patient has no signs of life (based on lack of purposeful movement, normal breathing, coughing) or there is any doubt, start CPR (step 4B) until more help arrives or the patient shows signs of life.

Figure 3.10 Assess for breathing and signs of life

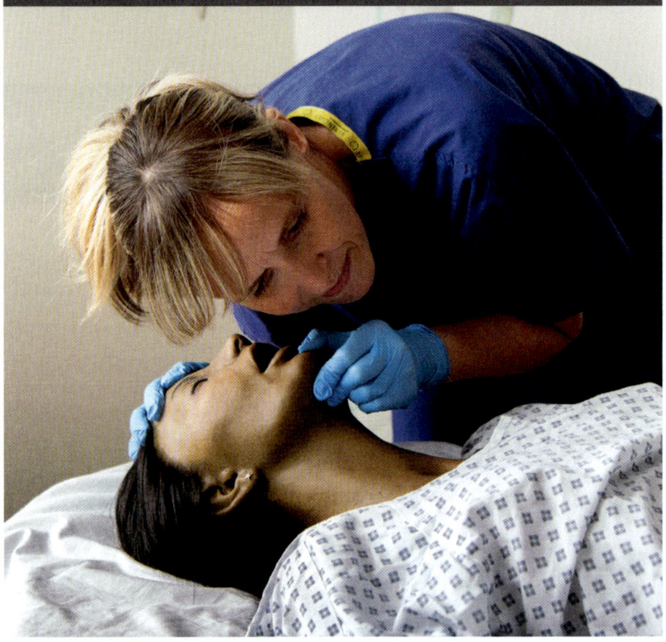

Diagnosing cardiac arrest can be difficult. If unsure, do not delay starting CPR. The patient is far more likely to die if there is a delay diagnosing cardiac arrest and starting CPR. Starting CPR on a very sick patient with a low blood pressure is unlikely to be harmful and may help. Assess the patient to confirm cardiac arrest even if the patient is monitored in a critical care area.

4A. If they have a pulse or other signs of life

Urgent clinical assessment is required. Depending on the local procedures, this may take the form of a resuscitation team or paramedics.

- Call for help.
- While waiting for the team, assess the patient using the ABCDE assessment (Chapter 2).

  A B C D E
- Give oxygen.
- Attach monitoring.
- Insert an intravenous cannula.
- The patient is at high risk of further deterioration and cardiac arrest and needs continued observation until the team arrives.

4A. If there are NO signs of life and NO pulse

- Start CPR.
- As appropriate, get a colleague to call the resuscitation team, call 999 for the ambulance service or for out-of-hospital providers, request additional resources to support (Figure 3.12) and collect the resuscitation equipment and a defibrillator.
- If alone, leave the patient to get help and equipment.
- Give 30 chest compressions followed by 2 ventilations.
- The correct hand position for chest compression is the middle of the lower half of the sternum. Place the heel of one hand in the centre of the chest with the other hand on top (Figure 3.13).
- Ensure high-quality chest compressions:
  - depth of 5–6 cm
  - rate of 100–120 compressions per min
  - allow the chest to recoil completely after each compression
  - take approximately the same amount of time for compression and recoil
  - minimise any interruptions to chest compression (hands-off time).
- If available, use a prompt and/or feedback device to help ensure high-quality chest compressions. Do not feel for pulses to assess the effectiveness of chest compressions.
- Each time compressions are resumed, place your hands without delay in the centre of the chest.
- The person doing chest compressions will get tired. If there are enough rescuers, this person should change about every 2 minutes or earlier if unable to maintain high-quality chest compressions. Plan ahead to ensure this change is done with minimal interruption to compressions, e.g. swap CPR provider during planned pauses in chest compression during rhythm assessment.
- Use whatever equipment is available immediately for airway and ventilation; for example, a pocket mask with an oral airway adjunct and oxygen, or a two-person self-inflating bag-valve mask (Figure 3.14), or a supraglottic airway (e.g. laryngeal mask airway (LMA) or i-gel) and bag-valve device. In practice, patients can have several airway techniques used stepwise during a cardiac arrest as equipment arrives and according to the skills of the rescuer (Chapter 9).

Figure 3.12 Responder call 2222 for cardiac arrest team / Community hospitals call 999 for ambulance

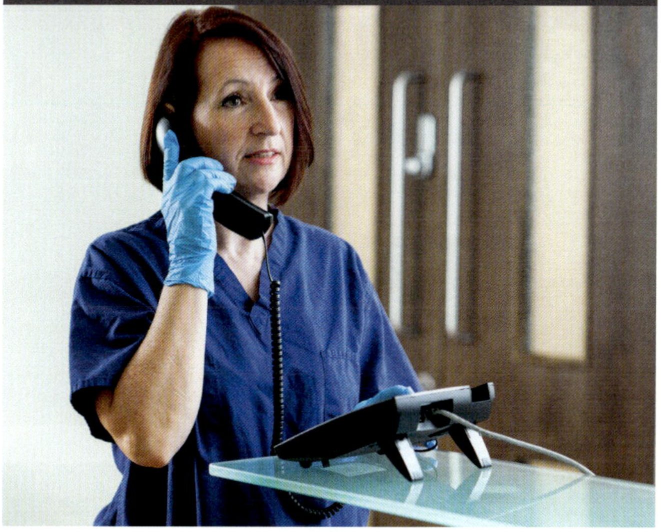

Figure 3.13 Hand position for chest compressions

Place the heel of one hand in the centre of the chest with the other hand on top

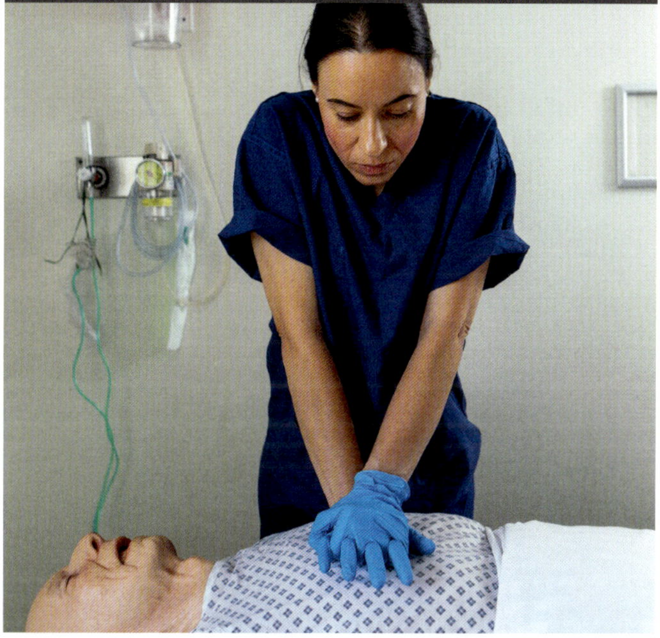

Figure 3.14 Two-person bag-mask ventilation during 30:2 CPR

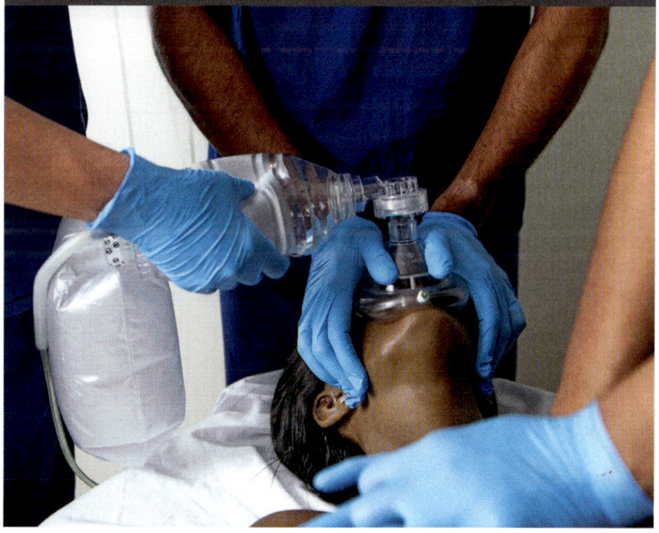

Figure 3.15 Maintain chest compressions while self-adhesive pads are applied

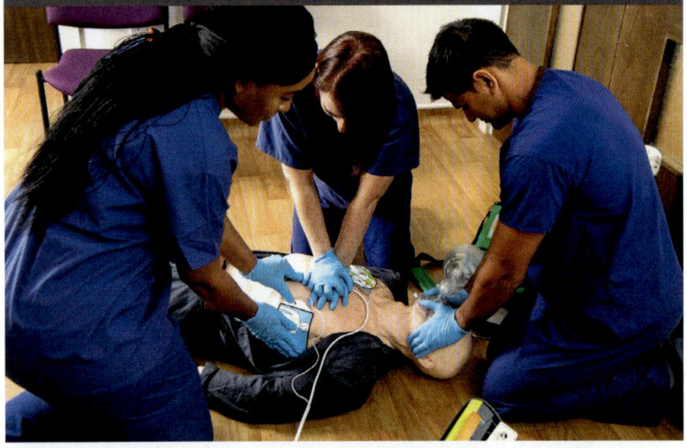

Figure 3.16 Stopping to check the rhythm

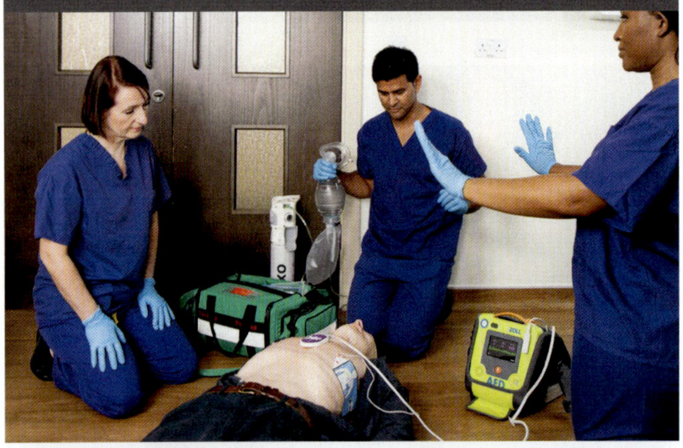

Figure 3.17 Push the shock button as directed by AED

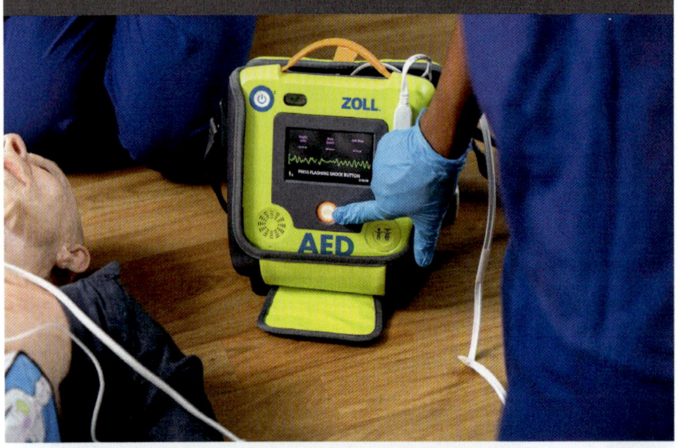

Figure 3.18 Resume CPR as prompted by AED

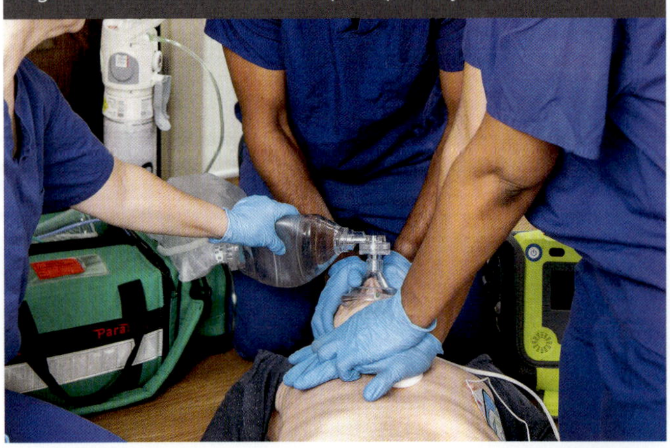

- If airway and ventilation equipment are unavailable, consider mouth-to-mouth ventilation. If there are clinical reasons to avoid mouth-to-mouth contact, or you are unable to do this, do chest compression-only CPR until help or airway equipment arrives. There are usually good clinical reasons to avoid mouth-to-mouth ventilation in clinical settings, and it is therefore rarely used, but there will be situations where giving mouth-to-mouth breaths could be lifesaving. A pocket mask or bag-valve mask should be immediately available in all clinical areas. A pocket mask with a filter, or a barrier device with a one-way valve, will minimise infection risk during rescue breathing.

- Irrespective of how you ventilate the patient's lungs, use an inspiratory time of about 1 second and give enough volume to produce a visible rise of the chest wall. Add supplemental oxygen as soon as possible. Avoid rapid or forceful breaths and overinflation.

- Insertion of a supraglottic airway or tracheal intubation should be attempted only by those who are trained, competent and experienced, and who can insert the tracheal tube/supraglottic device with minimal interruption (less than 5 seconds) to chest compressions.

- Waveform capnography must be used routinely for confirming that a tracheal tube is in the patient's airway and for subsequent monitoring during CPR. Once the patient's trachea has been intubated, continue chest compressions uninterrupted (except for defibrillation or pulse checks when indicated), at a rate of 100–120 min^{-1}, and ventilate the lungs at approximately 10 breaths min^{-1} (i.e. do not stop chest compressions for ventilation). If a supraglottic airway (e.g. LMA or i-gel) device has been inserted, it may also be possible to ventilate the patient's lungs without stopping chest compressions.

AED defibrillation

1. Switch on the AED and attach the electrode pads.

2. If more than one rescuer is present, continue chest compressions uninterrupted whilst the defibrillator pads are attached (Figure 3.15).

3. Follow the voice/visual directions.

4. Ensure that nobody touches the individual while the AED is analysing the rhythm (Figure 3.16). Some newer AEDs have the ability to analyse the rhythm during chest compressions. Follow instructions from the AED.

If a shock IS indicated:

5. Ensure that nobody touches the individual.
6. Push the shock button as directed (Figure 3.17).
7. Immediately resume CPR.

If a shock is NOT indicated:

8. Immediately resume CPR as prompted by the AED if no signs of life (Figure 3.18). There will be a period of CPR (2 minutes) before the AED prompts for a further pause in CPR for rhythm analysis.

Manual defibrillation

If trained and confident in rhythm recognition, use a manual defibrillator:

1. Perform uninterrupted chest compressions while applying self-adhesive defibrillation/monitoring pads as described above (Figure 3.15).
2. Plan actions before pausing CPR for rhythm analysis and communicate these to the team.
3. Stop chest compressions; confirm VF/pVT from the ECG. Ensure that this pause in chest compressions is brief and no longer than 5 seconds.
4. Resume chest compressions immediately; warn all rescuers other than the individual performing the chest compressions to "stand clear" (Figure 3.19) and remove any oxygen delivery device as appropriate, e.g. bag-valve-mask.
5. The designated person selects the appropriate energy on the defibrillator and presses the charge button. Choose an energy setting of 120 to 150 J for the first shock, the same or a higher energy for subsequent shocks, or follow the manufacturer's guidance for the particular defibrillator.
6. Ensure that the rescuer giving the compressions is the only person touching the patient.
7. Once the defibrillator is charged and the safety check is complete, tell the rescuer doing the chest compressions to "stand clear" (Figure 3.20); when clear, give the shock.
8. After shock delivery, immediately restart CPR, starting with chest compressions (Figure 3.21).
9. Do not pause to reassess the rhythm or feel for a pulse. Continue CPR for 2 minutes; the team leader prepares the team for the next pause in CPR.

Figure 3.19 No one is touching the patient during shock delivery

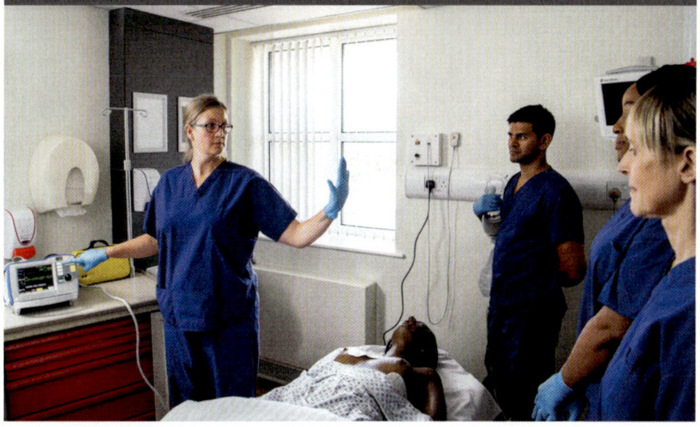

Figure 3.20 Stand clear

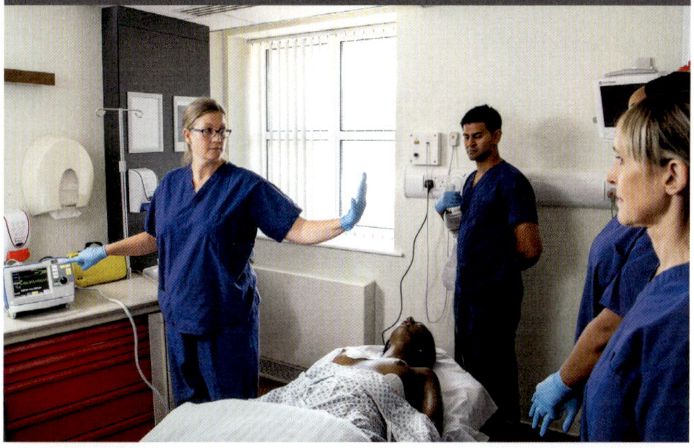

Figure 3.21 Immediately restart CPR using 30:2 ratio

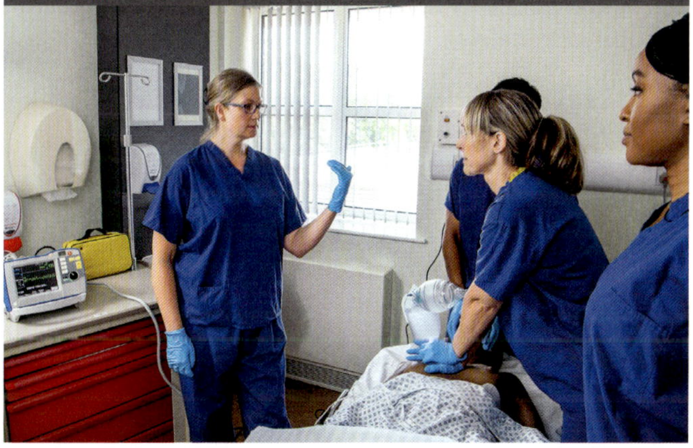

Figure 3.22 Chest compressions until team arrives

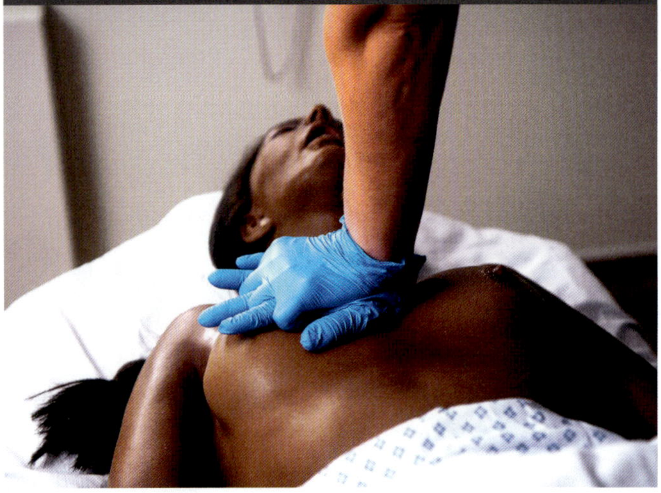

Figure 3.23 Ventilate

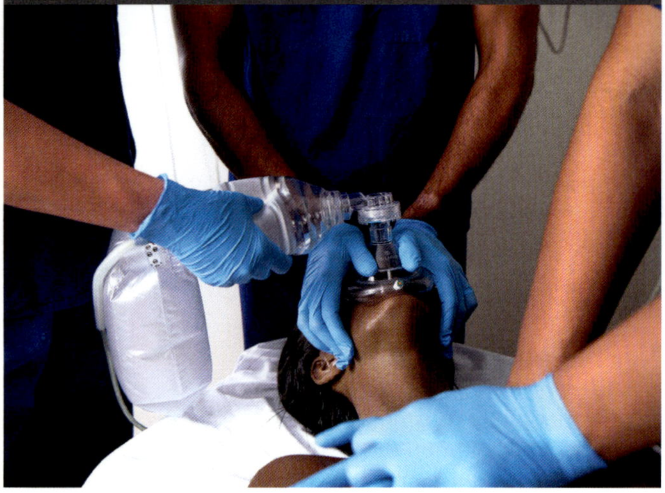

10. Pause briefly to check the monitor. This pause in chest compressions should be brief and no longer than 5 seconds.
11. If VF/pVT, repeat steps 3–10 above and deliver a second shock.
12. When using a manual defibrillator, further treatments will depend on the cardiac arrest rhythm.
13. See Chapter 8 for treatment of the different cardiac arrest rhythms.

ALL resuscitation attempts

- Continue resuscitation until further help arrives or the patient shows signs of life.
- Once resuscitation is underway, and if there are sufficient staff present, prepare intravenous cannulae and drugs likely to be used by the resuscitation team (e.g. adrenaline).
- Use a clock for timing between rhythm checks. It is difficult to keep track of the number of 30:2 cycles. In practice, rhythm checks should be performed every 2 minutes (AEDs will automatically time the 2-minute interval between rhythm check prompts). Some manual defibrillators will display a countdown timer on the screen.
- Make every effort to ensure that continuous, effective chest compressions are maintained throughout the resuscitation attempt. The importance of uninterrupted chest compressions cannot be overemphasised. Even brief interruptions to chest compressions can negatively affect the outcome.
- Plan exactly what you are going to do before stopping compressions to minimise the duration of the pause in compressions. Identify one person to be responsible for handover to the resuscitation team leader. Use SBARD or RSVP for handover (Table 4.1). Locate the patient's records.

4C. If they are NOT breathing and HAVE a pulse (respiratory arrest)

- Ventilate the patient's lungs using an inspiratory time of about 1 second and give enough volume to produce a visible rise of the chest wall. Check for a pulse every 10 breaths (about every minute).
- This diagnosis can be made only if you are confident in assessing breathing and pulse, and the patient has other signs of life.
- If there are any doubts about the presence of a pulse, start chest compressions until more experienced help arrives.
- All patients in respiratory arrest will develop cardiac arrest if the respiratory arrest is not treated rapidly and effectively.

03 SUMMARY LEARNING

Check for responsiveness, regular breathing, and signs of life to confirm cardiac arrest. This should take less than 10 seconds. Call for help and start CPR with chest compressions.

Deliver high-quality chest compressions with a depth of 5–6 cm, rate of 100–120 min^{-1}.

Minimise interruptions to chest compressions for other interventions, including defibrillation – this means all interruptions must be planned before stopping compressions.

For the patient in VF/pVT, early defibrillation is the only effective means of restoring a spontaneous circulation.

Use an AED if you are not confident in rhythm recognition or manual defibrillation.

TEST YOURSELF QUESTIONS

1. What number should you call for help following recognition of a cardiac arrest in your clinical setting?
2. What is the correct hand position for chest compression?
3. How quickly should defibrillation be attempted?

Further reading

Drennan IR, Greif R, Bray JE, et al., on behalf of the ILCOR Advanced Life Support Task Force. 2025 International Consensus on Cardiopulmonary Resuscitation and Emergency Cardiovascular Care Science With Treatment Recommendations. Advanced Life Support. ILCOR, 2025. In print.

Intensive Care National Audit & Research Centre (2024) National Cardiac Arrest Audit: Summary Statistics 2022–23. London: ICNARC. Available at: https://www.icnarc.org/wp-content/uploads/2024/05/NCAA-Summary-Statistics-2022-23.pdf.pdf (Accessed: 10 July 2025).

Smyth M, van Goor S, Giuseppe Ristagno, Malta Hansen C. et al. European Resuscitation Council 2025: Basic Life Support. Resuscitation. 2025. In print.

Soar J, Böttiger B, Carli P, et al. European Resuscitation Council Guidelines 2025: Advanced Life Support. Resuscitation. 2025.In print.

Vaillancourt C, Olasveengen TM, Bray JE, et al., on behalf of the ILCOR Basic Life Support Task Force. 2025 International Consensus on Cardiopulmonary Resuscitation and Emergency Cardiovascular Care Science With Treatment Recommendations. Basic Life Support. ILCOR, 2025. In print.

My key take-home messages from this chapter are:

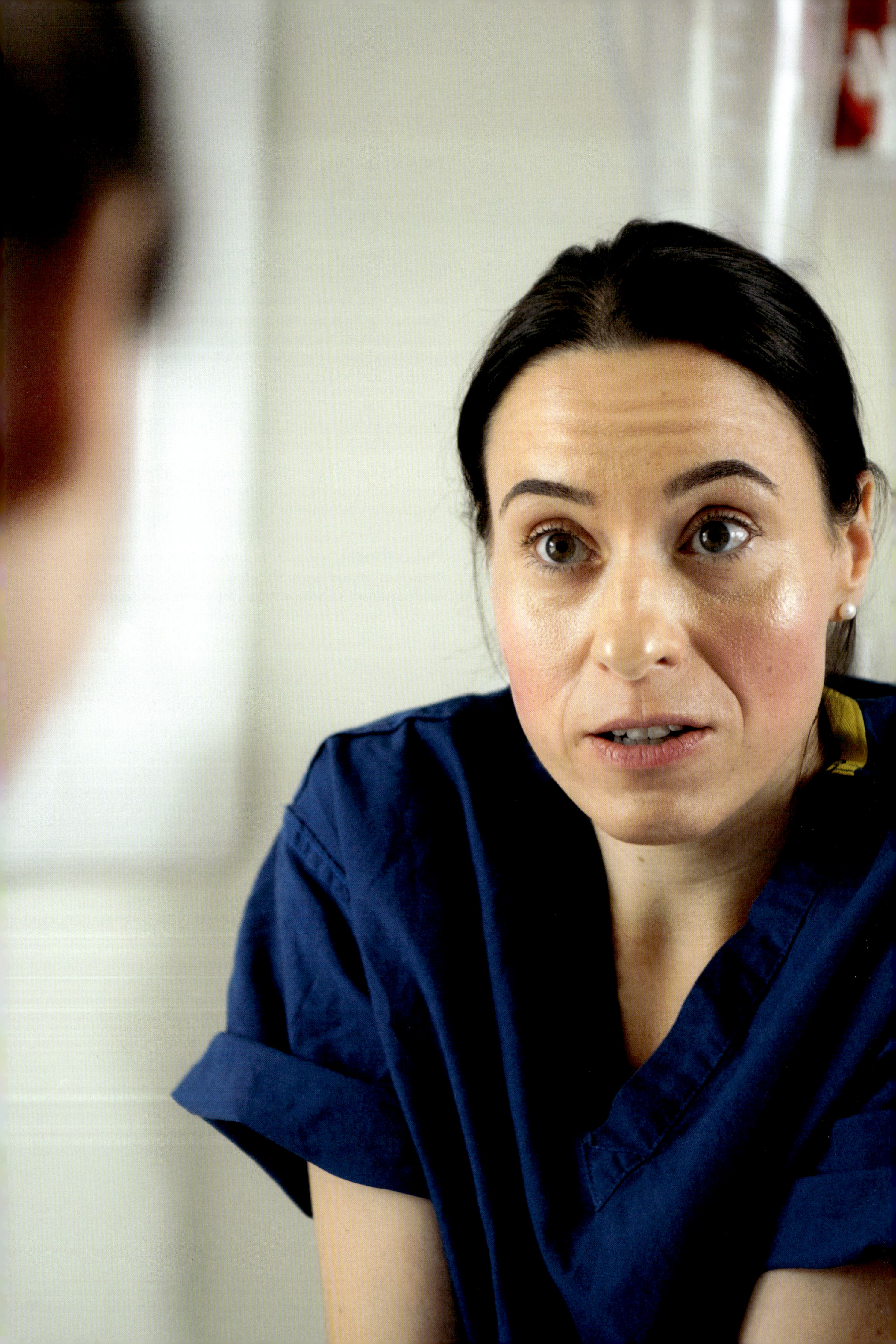

04 Non-technical skills in resuscitation

In this chapter

Non-technical skills:
- Situational awareness
- Decision making
- Team working (including leadership)
- Workload management

The importance of communication in resuscitation teams

The learning outcomes will enable you to:

Start immediate resuscitation

Be an effective team leader and team member

Consider the role of non-technical skills during resuscitation

Effectively use structured communication tools such as SBARD and RSVP

Introduction

The skills of chest compressions, defibrillation, and rhythm recognition are typically considered to be important aspects of cardiac arrest management. These are all technical skills that are learnt from books, lectures, courses and peers. Although they are important for the successful resuscitation of a patient, there is another group of important skills called non-technical skills.

Non-technical skills can be defined as the cognitive, social and personal resource skills that complement technical skills and contribute to safe and efficient task performance. More simply, they are the things that affect our personal performance. Non-technical skills of leadership and teamwork have been identified as important contributory factors to technical skill performance. Suboptimal leadership and teamworking have been identified as significant contributory factors resulting in poor clinical outcomes in both simulated and acute medical settings.

The importance of non-technical skills in emergencies is now widely accepted across many acute specialties. Examples of deficits include unwillingness to help, ineffective communication, weak leadership, suboptimal decision making, and unclear role allocation, all of which can lead to system errors. Episodes of cardiac arrest with documented system errors are associated with poor clinical outcomes such as decreased rates of return of spontaneous circulation and reduced survival rates. In the context of resuscitation, which is fundamentally a team effort, the contribution of teamwork and leadership is therefore expected to make a significant contribution to patient outcome.

Previous research has demonstrated that high-performing leadership behaviour is correlated with quality of CPR, with shorter hands-off time, pre-shock pauses and time to first shock. Understanding and improving non-technical skills may help with reducing human errors, creating more effective teams and improving patient safety. An effective team leader can help focus the team members, improve team commitment and act as the role model for the others.

The key non-technical skills are:

- situational awareness
- decision-making
- leadership and team working
- workload management
- communication.

Situational awareness

This can be described as an individual's awareness of the environment at the moment of an event and the analysis of this to understand how an individual's actions may impact on future events. This becomes particularly important when many events are happening simultaneously, for example, at a cardiac arrest. High information input with poor situational awareness may lead to poor decision-making and serious consequences. During a cardiac arrest, all those participating will have varying degrees of situational awareness. In a well-functioning team, all members will have a common understanding of current events, or shared situational awareness. It is important that only the relevant information is shared; otherwise, there is too much distraction or noise.

Situational awareness in cardiac arrest will include perception of environment and events taking place, comprehension of their meaning, and future projection.

INFORMATION GATHERING
What are the potential causes of arrest?

- Location of arrest.
- Information from staff about events leading up to the arrest.
- Note the actions already initiated.
- Confirm who is present – names, skills, roles and who is leading.

INTERPRETATION
What immediate steps are needed?

- Confirm diagnosis/cardiac arrest.
- Checking that a monitor has been attached and interpreting the rhythm.
- Determine immediate needs and necessary actions.

FUTURE PLANNING
What are the next steps?

- Consider the impact of interventions.
- Plan for next steps.

Decision-making

This is defined as the cognitive process of choosing a specific course of action from several alternatives. During a cardiac arrest, the many decisions to be made usually fall to the team leader. The leader will assimilate information from the team members and from personal observation and will use this to determine appropriate interventions.

Typical decisions made at a cardiac arrest include:

- Choice of shock energy to be used for defibrillation.
- Likely reversible causes of the cardiac arrest.
- Appropriate treatment such as drugs or airway management.
- How long to continue resuscitation.
- Appropriate post-resuscitation care.

Once a decision has been made, clear, unambiguous communication with the team members is essential to ensure that it is implemented.

Team working, including team leadership

This is one of the most important non-technical skills that contributes to successful management of critical situations. A team is a group of individuals working together with a common goal or purpose. In a team, the members usually have complementary skills and, through coordination of effort, work synergistically. Teams work best when everyone knows each other's name, when they are doing something they perceive to be important, and when their role is within their experience and competence. There are several characteristics of a good resuscitation team member:

Competence – has the skills required at a cardiac arrest and performs them to the best of their ability.

Commitment – strives to achieve the best outcome for the patient.

Communicates openly – being able to articulate their findings and actions taken, raise concerns about clinical or safety issues, listens to briefings and instructions and practices effective closed loop communication.

Supportive – enables others to achieve their best.

Accountable – for their own and the team's actions

Prepared to admit when help is needed.

Creative – suggests different ways of interpreting the situation.

Participates in providing feedback.

Figure 4.1 Team leader using a checklist

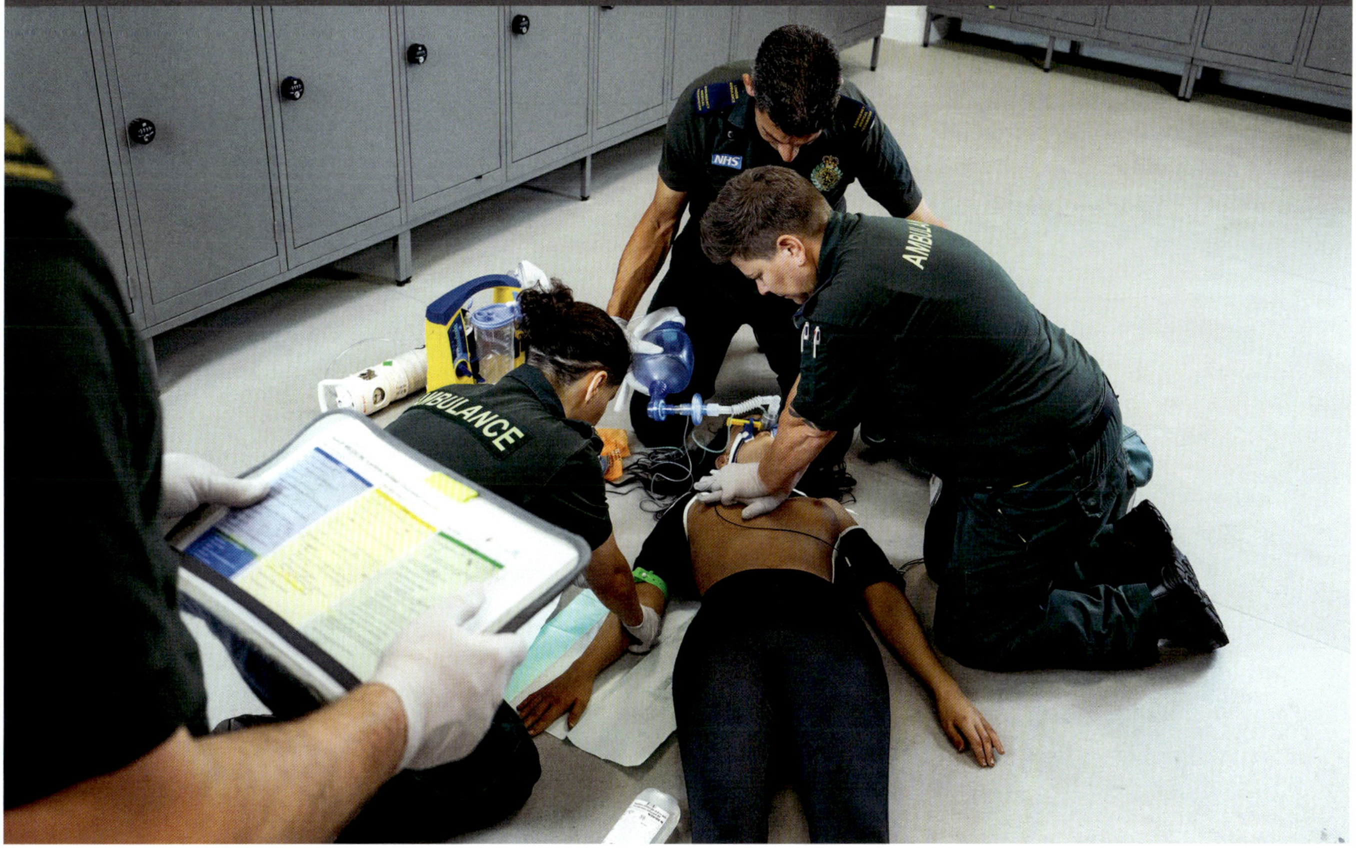

Team leadership

Optimal team function mandates a team leader. A team leader provides guidance, direction and instruction to the team members to enable successful completion of their stated objective (Figure 4.1). They lead by example and integrity. Team leaders need experience, not simply seniority. Team leadership can be considered a process; it is available to everyone with training, role modelling and support. There are several attributes recognisable in a good team leader:

- Knows everyone in the team by name and knows their capability.
- Accepts the leadership role.
- Is able to delegate tasks appropriately.
- Is knowledgeable and has sufficient credibility to influence the team through role-modelling and professionalism.
- Recognises their own limitations and asks for support from the team.
- Is a good communicator – provides clarity when giving instructions, is a good listener and decisive in action.
- Stays calm, keeps everyone focused and manages distractions.
- Is empathetic towards the whole team using emotional intelligence.
- Is assertive and authoritative when required.
- Shows tolerance towards hesitancy or nervousness in the emergency setting.
- Has good situational awareness; able to constantly monitor the situation, with an up-to-date overview, listening and deciding on a course of action.

During a cardiac arrest, the role of team leader is not always immediately obvious. The leader should state early on that they are assuming the role of team leader.

Specifically, at a cardiac arrest the leader should:

- Follow current resuscitation guidelines or explain a reason for any significant deviation from standard protocols.
- Consult with the team or call for senior advice and assistance if unsure about an intervention.
- Play to the strengths of team members and allow them some autonomy if their skills are adequate.
- Allocate roles and tasks throughout the resuscitation and be specific. This avoids several people or nobody attempting the task.
- Use the 2-minute periods of chest compressions to plan tasks and consider safety aspects of the resuscitation attempt with the team.
- Thank the team at the end of the resuscitation attempt and ensure that staff and relatives are being supported.
- Complete all documentation and ensure an adequate handover.

Table 4.1 SBARD (Situation, Background, Assessment, Recommendation, Decision) **and RSVP** (Reason, Story, Vital signs, Plan)

SBARD	RSVP	Content	Example
Situation	**Reason**	Introduce yourself and check you are speaking to the correct person. Identify the patient you are calling about (who and where). Say what you think the current problem is, or appears to be. State what you need advice about. Useful phrases: • The problem appears to be cardiac/ respiratory/neurological/sepsis. • I'm not sure what the problem is but the patient is deteriorating. • The patient is unstable, getting worse and I need help.	Hi, I'm Dr Bradfield the medical F2. I am calling about Mr Grafton on acute medical admissions who I think has a severe pneumonia and is septic. He has an oxygen saturation of 90% despite high-flow oxygen and I am very worried about him.
Background	**Story**	Background information about the patient. Reason for admission. Relevant past medical history.	He is 55 and previously fit and well. He has had fever and a cough for 2 days. He arrived 30 minutes ago by ambulance.
Assessment	**Vital signs**	Include specific observations and vital sign values based on the ABCDE assessment. • Airway • Breathing • Circulation • Disability • Exposure • The early warning score is…	He looks very unwell and is tiring. Airway – he can say a few words. Breathing – his respiratory rate is 24, he has bronchial breathing on the left side. His oxygen saturation is 90% on high-flow oxygen. I am getting a blood gas and chest X-ray. Circulation – his pulse is 110, his blood pressure is 110/60. Disability – he is drowsy but can say a few words. Exposure – he has no rashes.
Recommendation	**Plan**	State explicitly what you want the person you are calling to do. What by when? Useful phrases: • I am going to start the following treatment; is there anything else you can suggest? • I am going to do the following investigations; is there anything else you can suggest? • If they do not improve; when would you like to be called? • I don't think I can do anymore; I would like you to see the patient urgently.	I am getting antibiotics ready and he is on IV fluids. I need help – please can you come and see him straight away.
Decision		Summarise what has been agreed. Confirm what has been discussed.	We have agreed that you will come and review the patient straight away. In the meantime I will repeat the BP reading.

Workload management

During the resuscitation of a patient, either in cardiac arrest or peri-arrest, there are numerous tasks to be carried out by the team members, either sequentially or simultaneously. Cognitive aids such as checklists or easy-access guidelines could be used as support but will need a dedicated team member to read and check. The coordination and control, or management, of these tasks is the responsibility of the team leader (Figure 4.2).

Tasks can include:

- Planning and, where appropriate, briefing of the team (e.g. prior to arrival of the patient in the emergency department).
- Identifying the resources required – ensuring that equipment is checked and specifics organised and delegated.
- Being inclusive of all team members.
- Being prepared for both the expected and the unexpected.
- Prioritising actions of the team.
- Watching out for fatigue, stress and distress amongst the team.
- Managing conflict.
- Communicating with relatives.
- Communicating with experts for safe handover both by telephone and in person.
- Debriefing the team.
- Reporting untoward incidents, particularly equipment or system failures.
- Participation in audit (Chapter 1).

The importance of communication when managing a sick patient

Communication problems contribute to up to 80% of adverse events and near misses in acute hospitals, particularly during handovers, and can also occur in community and out-of-hospital teams, both between each other and at the point of care transfer.

This is especially evident during emergency situation when a clinician summons senior help. Unstructured calls can obscure the seriousness of the situation, omit key facts and fail to convey urgency. Incomplete or ambiguous information can also heighten the responder's anxiety and leave them uncertain about what they are about to face.

Using a simple, reliable structure, for example SBARD, enables the caller to communicate the essentials and urgency, and helps the recipient plan ahead. The same rationale underpins the ABCDE approach, an aide-mémoire that structures assessment and management of the acutely unwell and peri-arrest patient.

The use of the SBARD (Situation, Background, Assessment, Recommendation, Decisions) or RSVP (Reason, Story, Vital signs, Plan) tools enables effective, timely communication between individuals from different clinical backgrounds and hierarchies (Table 4.1).

Figure 4.2 Team leader prioritising actions of the team

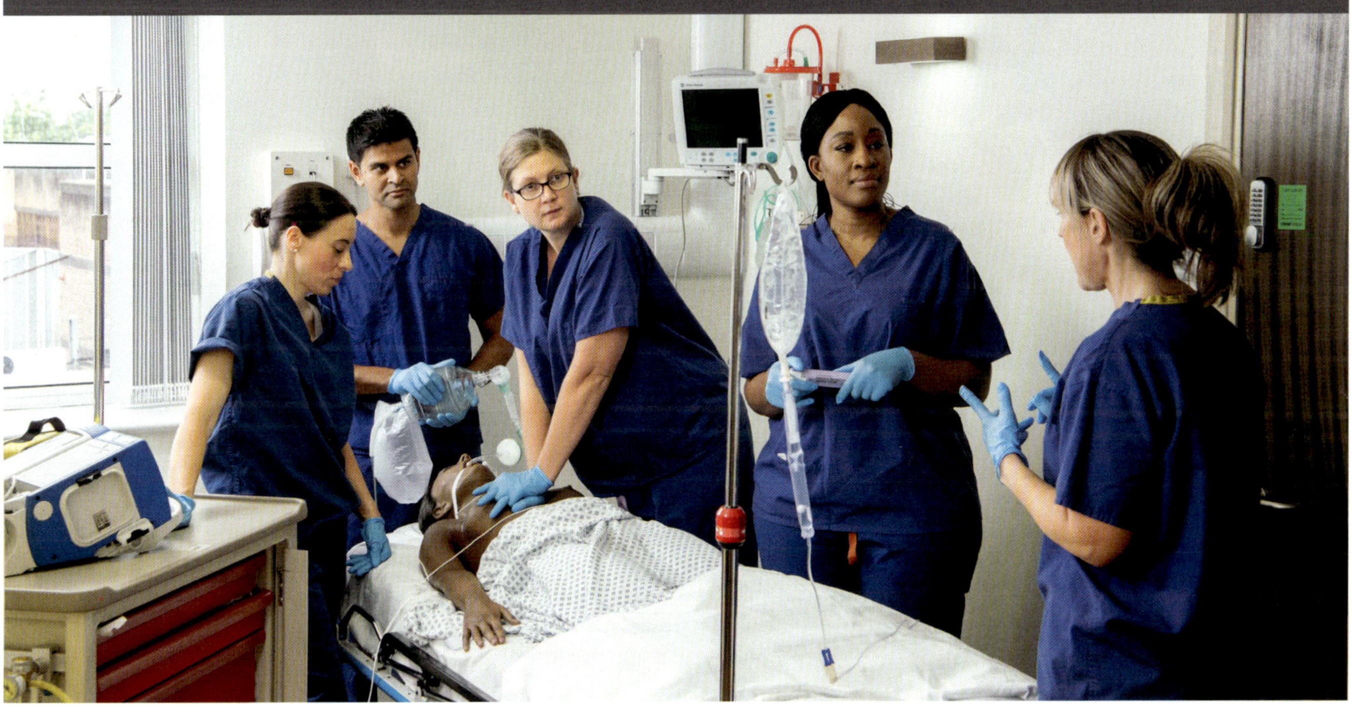

Resuscitation teams

The resuscitation team is a generic term and is reflective of the dynamic nature of team formation as the team may change daily or more frequently. As a result of shift pattern working in hospital, or out-of-hospital responders tasked to an incident by their proximity at the point of call, members may not know each other or the skill mix of the team members.

Where possible, team should therefore meet at the beginning of their period on duty to:

- Introduce themselves; communication is much easier and more effective if people can be referred to by their name.
- Identify everyone's skills and experience.
- Allocate the team leader. Skill and experience take precedence over seniority.
- Allocate responsibilities; if key skills are lacking (e.g. advanced airway management), work out how this deficit can be managed (Figure 4.3).
- Review any patients who have been identified as 'at risk' during the previous duty period.

SCAN ME for responder wellbeing support

Finally, every effort should be made to enable the team members to meet and debrief in a psychologically safe environment. This allows the opportunity to openly explore difficulties or concerns about performance, issues with equipment and consider the need to submit an incident report).

Resuscitation Council UK has developed an on-line resource: Rescuer Wellbeing – available at www.resus.org.uk/responder-wellbeing.

Figure 4.3 Team brief / debrief

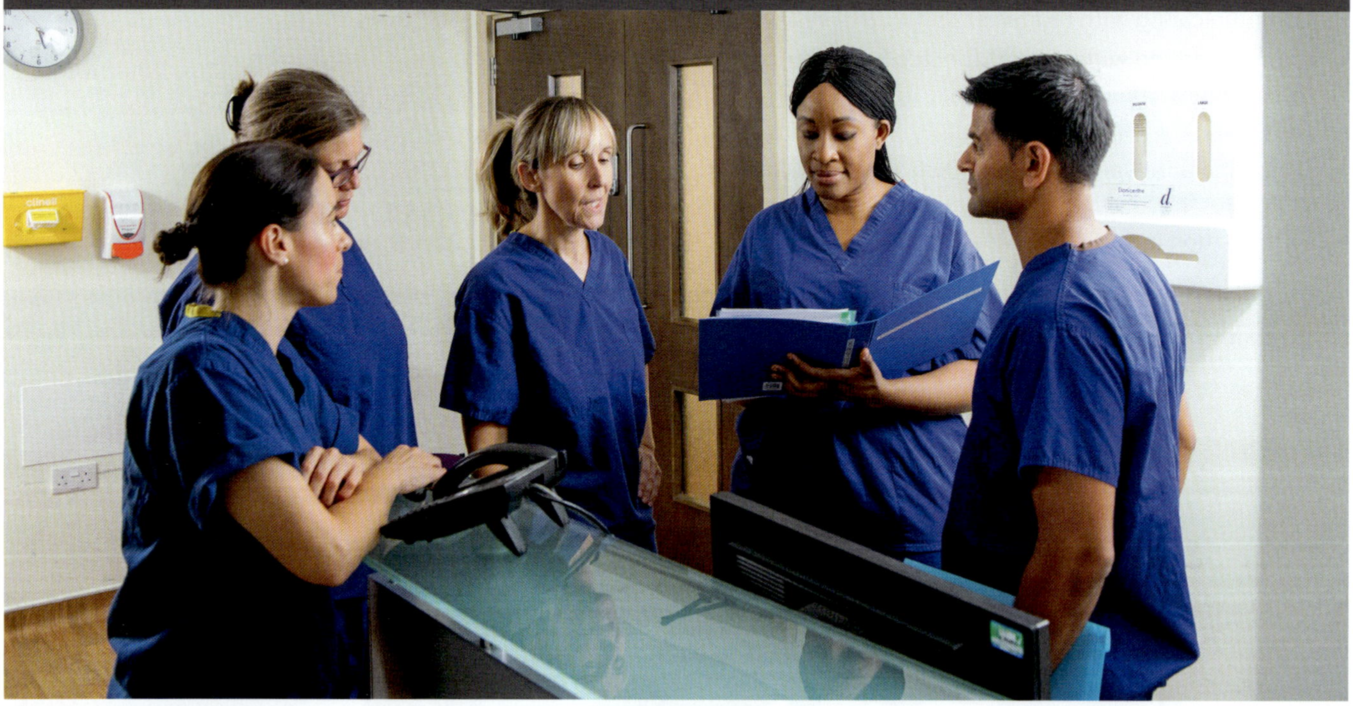

04 SUMMARY LEARNING

Non-technical skills are important during resuscitation.

Use SBARD or RSVP for effective communication.

TEST YOURSELF QUESTIONS

1. What does the communication tool SBARD stand for?
2. Can you name some of the activities that resuscitation team members can do to improve teamwork if they meet at the beginning of a period of duty?

Further reading

Andersen PO, Jensen MK, Lippert A, et al: Identifying non-technical skills and barriers for improvement of teamwork in cardiac arrest teams. Resuscitation 2010; 81:695–702.

Cooper SJ, Cant RP. Measuring non-technical skills of medical emergency teams: an update on the validity and reliability of the Team Emergency Assessment Measure (TEAM). Resuscitation. 2014;85(1):31-3.

Featherstone P, Chalmers T, Smith GB. RSVP: a system for communication of deterioration in hospital patients. Br J Nurs 2008;17:860-64.

Peltonen V, Peltonen LM, Salantera S et al. An observational study of technical and non-technical skills in advanced life support in the clinical setting. Resuscitation 2020; 53:162-168.

Yeung J, Ong G, Davies R, Gao F, Perkins GDP. Factors affecting team leadership skills and their relationship with quality of cardiopulmonary resuscitation. Crit Care Med 2012; 40:2617–2621.

Liu CH, Yang CW, Lockey A, Greif R, Cheng A; Education, Implementation, Team Task Force of the International Liaison Committee on Resuscitation ILCOR. Factors influencing workload and stress during resuscitation - A scoping review. Resusc Plus. 2024 Apr 19;18:100630.

Farquharson B, Cortegiani A, Lauridsen KG, Yeung J, Greif R, Nabecker S; Education Implementation Team Task Force of the International Liaison Committee on Resuscitation ILCOR. Teaching team competencies within resuscitation training: A systematic review. Resusc Plus. 2024 Jun 18;19:100687.

My key take-home messages from this chapter are:

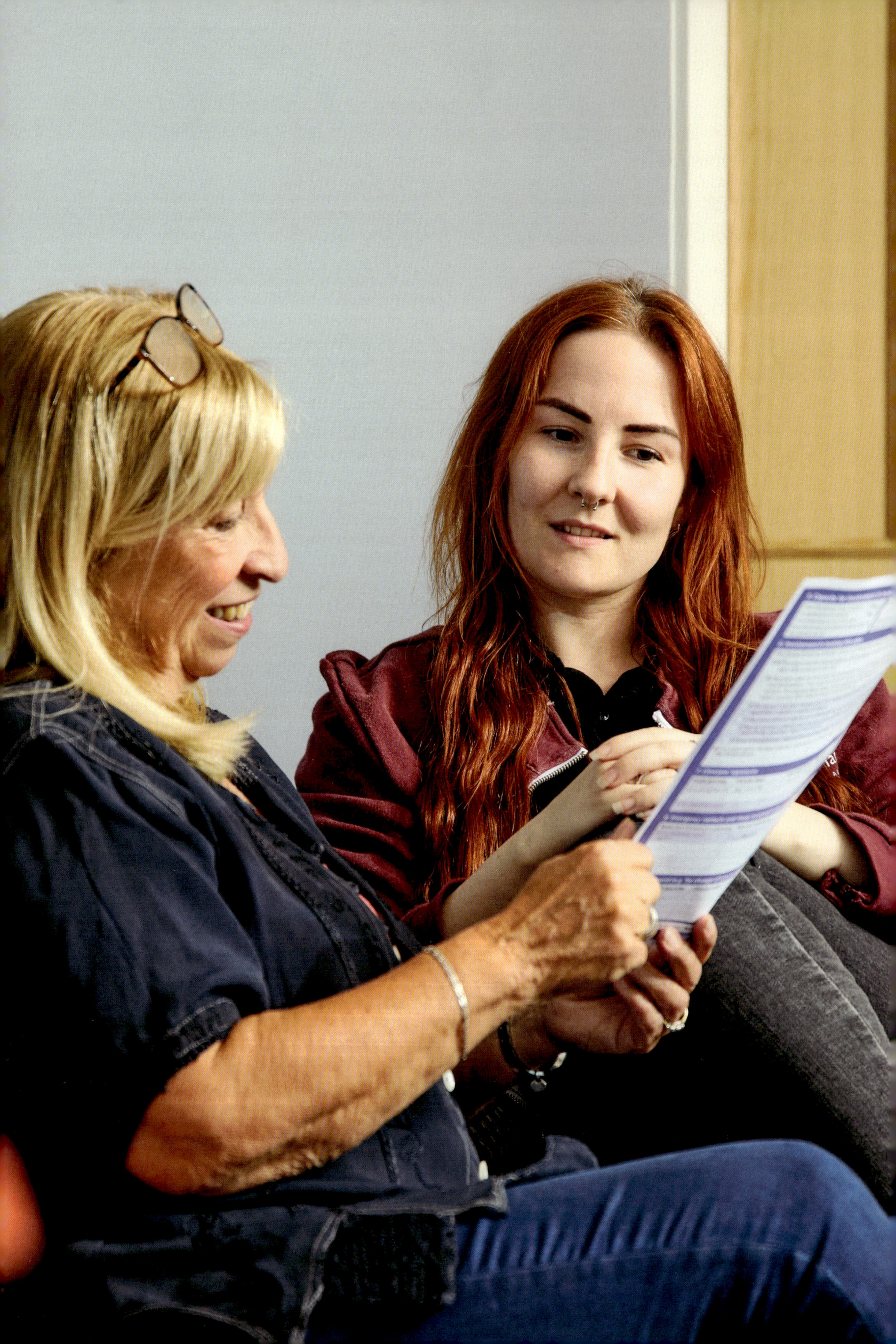

05 Decisions about CPR

In this chapter

Ethical and legal principles

Emergency care and treatment plans (including CPR)

Shared understanding and decision-making, effective communication and clear documentation

Deciding whether to provide CPR and deciding to stop CPR

Auditing cardiac arrest and recommendations and decisions about CPR

The learning outcomes will enable you to:

Consider the ethical and legal principles involved in providing recommendations and making decisions about emergency care and treatment, including CPR

Participate in shared decision-making to create personalised recommendations for a person's clinical care and treatment in a future emergency in which they are unable to make or express choices and involve those close to them where appropriate

Communicate effectively to elicit patient preferences, and explain what is realistic in terms of their care and treatment

Record clear and relevant information relating to emergency care treatment plans (including CPR)

Understand when it is reasonable to not attempt or discontinue CPR

Feel confident in reaching a shared understanding and decisions about emergency care and treatments, and encourage others to follow best practice

Introduction

Cardiopulmonary resuscitation (CPR) can be a lifesaving intervention bringing extended life to many. However, it is far from being universally successful and, like any invasive medical treatment, can cause harm.

When someone is dying from an irreversible cause, CPR is unlikely to work and can subject them to an undignified death, or even cause suffering and prolong the process of dying. Do not assume that everyone whose heart and breathing stop would consider survival a successful outcome. Prolonging life at all costs is not an appropriate goal of medicine.

Do not attempt CPR (DNACPR) decisions have existed for many years and provide a mechanism to not attempt CPR when it will not restart the heart or breathing for a sustained period, where the balance of burdens exceeds the benefits or the patient does not wish to receive CPR.

CPR is not provided in isolation from other treatments and should always be considered as part of an overall emergency care treatment plan

The Recommended Summary Plan for Emergency Care and Treatment (ReSPECT) process provides a framework to enable shared understanding and decision-making in relation to emergency treatment decisions (including CPR) when the person is unable to participate in decision-making at a future time. This chapter summarises the legal and ethical considerations for making such recommendations and describes how to engage patients and their families in shared decision-making.

The ReSPECT process is used across large parts of the UK but has not been universally adopted. Where the ResPECT process has not been adopted, local/regional processes should be used.

Ethical and legal framework

Healthcare professionals must practice ethically and within the law.

Laws relevant to CPR, including those on matters relating to capacity and consent, vary from nation to nation, both outside of and within the UK. Detailed guidance is provided in the 'Decisions relating to cardiopulmonary resuscitation' published by the RCUK, British Medical Association and Royal College of Nursing. The ethical and legal principles that underpin this guidance apply equally to the broader planning approach taken by the ReSPECT process and other emergency care and treatment plans. ILS providers should read and be familiar with that guidance, and relevant aspects of the law.

Table 5.1 summarises Beauchamp and Childress' four key principles of medical ethics, which is a commonly used framework for prompting consideration of ethical aspects of decision-making. Every decision about CPR must be based on a careful assessment of each person's situation at any particular time. These decisions must never be dictated by 'blanket' policies. Individual decisions about CPR must be made with the person, or where they lack capacity, with those close to them. The courts have made clear that there should be a presumption in favour of involving people in discussions about whether or not CPR will be attempted. This upholds the principle of autonomy and the provisions of the Human Rights Act (1998).

There are two rare circumstances where it is legally and ethically acceptable to make a CPR decision without discussion with the person or those close to them:

1. Where it is believed that having a conversation with the person will cause physiological or psychological harm to them (Tracey v Cambridge University Hospital).
2. In the case of a person who lacks capacity to make a decision regarding CPR, where it is impracticable or inappropriate to contact those close to them before a decision needs to be made (Winspear v City Hospitals). This would include, for example, emergencies where an individual had lost capacity and there was insufficient time to contact those close to them, or it was not possible to reach them.

Integrate recommendations relating to CPR in to overarching emergency care treatment plans

Research has shown that when DNACPR decisions are made in isolation they lack clarity on the overall goals of treatment.

In some cases, this has unintentionally led to fewer invasive medical treatments, reduced observations, less escalation to medical and outreach staff and reductions in even basic nursing care. The integration of decisions relating to CPR into overarching emergency care treatment plans has been shown to reduce harms, increase clarity of overall goals of care, improve concordance between a patient's wishes and treatments provided and enhance communication between clinicians and the patient. Therefore, it is recommended that decisions to provide or not to provide CPR should always be made in the context of an overall plan for emergency care and treatment.

Shared understanding and decision-making

Shared understanding and decision-making brings together the individual's expertise about themselves and what is important to them and the clinician's knowledge about the benefits and risks of relevant treatments.

Table 5.1 Summary of Beauchamp and Childress' four key principles of medical ethics

Autonomy	Requires people to be allowed and helped to make their own informed decisions, rather than having decisions made for them. A person with capacity must be adequately informed about the matter to be decided and free from undue pressure in making their decision.	Autonomy allows an informed person to make a choice, even if that choice is considered illogical or incorrect by others, including health professionals.
Beneficence	Involves provision of benefit to an individual, while balancing benefit and risks. Commonly this will involve attempting CPR for cardiac arrest. If CPR will offer no benefit or the risks clearly outweigh any likely benefit, it will mean not attempting CPR.	Beneficence also includes actions that benefit the wider community, such as providing a programme of public access defibrillation.
Non-maleficence	Means doing no harm. CPR should not be attempted in people in whom it will not succeed, where no benefit is likely but there will be a clear risk of doing harm.	
Justice	Requires spreading benefits and risks equally within a society. If CPR is provided, it should be available to all who may benefit from it. There should be no discrimination purely on the grounds of factors such as age or disability.	Justice does not imply an entitlement to expect or demand CPR for everyone. If limited resources are engaged in attempting CPR on people with no chance of benefit, those resources may not be available when needed by others who are likely to benefit.

Many people welcome the opportunity to discuss their wishes about care, treatments and health outcomes, once they realise that the purpose of the planning is to establish with their healthcare professionals which treatments they may benefit from. Health professionals are not obliged to offer or deliver treatments that they believe to be inappropriate. Even where treatment options are limited, seek to engage patients in shared decision-making using the steps described below.

1. Establish what the person thinks are the most relevant health conditions and develop a shared understanding of the prognosis of these conditions. Find out how the person feels about their current environment and state of health, and their views about the future.
2. Establish and record what the person thinks would matter most to them (values and fears) if they suddenly became less well, both in their daily lives and as a possible future emergency.
3. Having established what is most important to the person, agree upon and record what interventions will result in the desired outcomes and so are wanted, and which ones have little realistic chance of success, or a high probability of resulting in a feared outcome, and so are unwanted or would not work. This includes, but is not limited to a recommendation about CPR.

The ReSPECT process (Figure 5.1) was developed to support this structure of shared understanding and decision-making; however, whatever process you use try to make sure the conversation is not just about CPR but also about wider goals of care. This approach can make the conversation more positive and useful for both the person and the clinician.

Specific training in having these sensitive conversations can help health professionals to communicate effectively and to recognise that these conversations are important and are not necessarily difficult.

Explore your opportunities for such training as part of your professional development.

Requirements for effective communication include providing information in a format that the person can understand and checking that they have understood it. It may be necessary to have more than one conversation to reach a shared understanding and a decision. Offer opportunities for further discussion and be aware that people may change their minds if they wish to.

Don't force conversations on people who don't want them, but don't withhold them from those who do. Whenever possible, these conversations should be undertaken by health professionals who know the person well, but that may not be possible when they are needed by someone with an acute illness or injury and no previous advance plan.

Figure 5.1 Recommended Summary Plan for Emergency Care and Treatment (ReSPECT) process

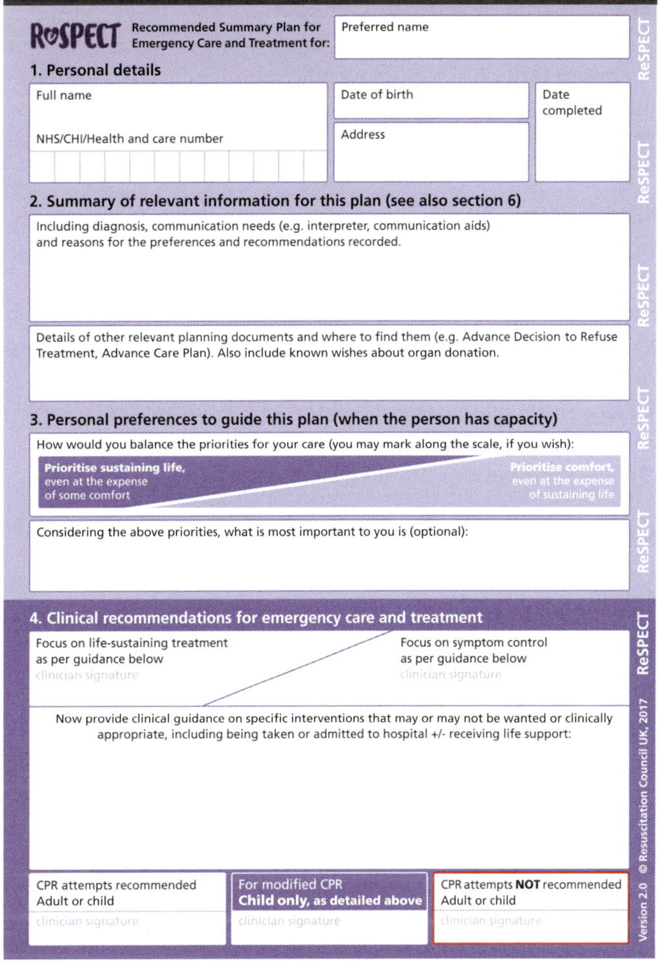
ReSPECT Recommended Summary Plan for Emergency Care and Treatment for:

Preferred name

1. Personal details

Full name

NHS/CHI/Health and care number

Date of birth

Address

Date completed

2. Summary of relevant information for this plan (see also section 6)

Including diagnosis, communication needs (e.g. interpreter, communication aids) and reasons for the preferences and recommendations recorded.

Details of other relevant planning documents and where to find them (e.g. Advance Decision to Refuse Treatment, Advance Care Plan). Also include known wishes about organ donation.

3. Personal preferences to guide this plan (when the person has capacity)

How would you balance the priorities for your care (you may mark along the scale, if you wish):

Prioritise sustaining life, even at the expense of some comfort

Prioritise comfort, even at the expense of sustaining life

Considering the above priorities, what is most important to you is (optional):

4. Clinical recommendations for emergency care and treatment

Focus on life-sustaining treatment as per guidance below

clinician signature

Focus on symptom control as per guidance below

clinician signature

Now provide clinical guidance on specific interventions that may or may not be wanted or clinically appropriate, including being taken or admitted to hospital +/- receiving life support:

CPR attempts recommended Adult or child

clinician signature

For modified CPR **Child only, as detailed above**

clinician signature

CPR attempts **NOT** recommended Adult or child

clinician signature

Version 2.0 © Resuscitation Council UK, 2017

Findings from an evaluation of ReSPECT, funded by the National Institute for Health Research, found that ReSPECT conversations take time for health professionals to do well.

Good decisions were characterised by building rapport and trust through:

- Exercising medical judgment when recommending certain treatments.
- Soliciting a person's view about their values and preferences.
- Taking these into account when making treatment recommendations.
- Talking a person through the rationale for these recommendations.
- Ensuring that decisions are understood.
- Recording how the harms and benefits associated with treatment options were weighed up.

Communication: discussing recommendations with those close to the person

An important component of high-quality care is effective communication with those close to a person (often, but not always, family members) and keeping them fully informed.

You must respect a person's wishes regarding confidentiality, but most people want family members or others close to them to be involved in discussions about treatments such as CPR and to have their support in making these decisions. Whenever possible, encourage patients to think about and discuss their wishes in advance with members of their family. Knowing a patient's wishes helps relatives to feel more confident in situations when they are asked what they think a patient would have wanted.

Communication: discussing recommendations when a person lacks capacity

In order for a person to be involved in a discussion about CPR or other emergency treatments, they need to have capacity to do so. This means that they must be able to understand, retain, weigh and communicate information about the situation and related decisions.

If a person lacks capacity, they can still be involved in decision-making to the limit of their ability. Formal assessment of their capacity should be undertaken and recorded in line with relevant local policy; remember that capacity is decision specific.

If a person does not have capacity to be involved in the discussions and recommendations being made, then decisions about their treatment, including about CPR, must be made according to capacity laws of the nation you are practising in.

If the patient has a legally binding document recording their refusal of specific treatments in given circumstances (e.g. an Advance Decision to Refuse Treatment in England and Wales), this must be adhered to by health professionals. Emergency care and treatment plans, such as ReSPECT and DNACPRs, are not legally binding; they provide recommendations to help aid decision making when an emergency occurs.

In all circumstances, those close to the patient need to be consulted so long as it is practicable and appropriate to do so.

Any conversation you have should follow the same structure provided above: establish a shared understanding of the person's condition, what is known of their wishes and fears, and what treatments, including CPR, that they would benefit from. The conversation should be fully documented.

If a person is critically ill and an urgent decision is needed in order to plan the best care for them, that decision should not be delayed if those close to them cannot be contacted. Make the decision that is in the person's best interests, using relevant policy and processes to support this, but also make and record a clear plan to consult their family, others close to them, or to contact an Independent Mental Capacity Advocate (in England and Wales), at the earliest practicable opportunity. Document the basis for any decision clearly and fully.

Providing recommendations about CPR

CPR should be recommended when it is likely to be of benefit to the person/patient.

CPR should not be recommended when:

- an informed person with capacity refuses it
- it would be unlikely to restart the heart and breathing for a sustained period because a person is dying as an inevitable result of underlying disease or a catastrophic health event.

A person (or someone representing them) is not entitled to insist on receiving a treatment that is clinically inappropriate. Healthcare professionals are not obliged to offer or deliver treatments that they believe to be inappropriate. Explaining these matters requires sensitive discussion. ReSPECT provides a suggested framework to help clinicians guide these conversations.

The overall responsibility for planning emergency care and treatment (including CPR) rests with the senior healthcare professional in charge of the person's care at the time. When making advance plans there should be appropriate consultation with other healthcare professionals involved, as well as appropriate discussion with the individual and those close to them.

If a difference of opinion arises between the healthcare team and the person or their representatives this can usually be resolved by careful discussion and explanation. This can include exploring and addressing any misconceptions about diagnosis, prognosis and treatment.

If disagreements persist, a second clinical opinion must be offered. Formal legal judgement accessed through an employing organisation may be needed if there are irreconcilable differences between the parties. In difficult cases, the senior clinician may wish to seek legal advice from their indemnity provider or other professional organisation.

When CPR attempts have not been recommended make sure that all other treatment is given in accordance with the person's treatment plan and is of the highest standard. This may include recording physiological observations, and treatments both at home and requiring transfer into hospital.

Recording emergency care and treatment plans (including CPR)

Ensure records include:

- Patient identifier information.
- Details of the person's health and current condition.
- What matters to the person and their priorities in decisions about their emergency care and treatment.
- Clinical recommendations for emergency care and treatment.
- Whether CPR should be attempted or not.
- Whether the person had mental capacity to be involved and their involvement in the recommendations that are being recorded.
- Others who were involved in the process.

Recommendations relating to emergency care and treatment (including CPR) should be recorded clearly and using terms that will be understandable to those who may need to act on them. Recommendations should be specific to the relevant treatments and also the setting where they may be applied.

Terms such as 'for ward based care' lack clarity on treatment goals and have limited relevance when someone is discharged from hosptial. Additionally, out-of-hospital clinicians may be accessing emergency care and treatment plans and may need make decisions about hospital conveyance.

Ensure the record is available immediately if it is needed in a crisis. For example, if such a recommendation is recorded on a paper form, this should be readily available to help an ambulance clinician decide whether to attempt CPR in a person's home. People should be encouraged and helped to make those close to them aware of what matters to them and resulting recommendations, and of where to find the record of these.

Various forms have been developed in different places to record people's treatment recommendations in advance. RCUK recommends use of the ReSPECT process and plan which is already accepted by many health and care provider organisations and can be used across geographical and organisational boundaries.

Communicating emergency care and treatment recommendations

There should be effective verbal communication with all those caring for the person and robust written and/or electronic documentation to ensure that recommendations are known, and the records remain available if the person travels to a different location, however briefly.

Within a hospital, that might involve, for example, attending a radiology or physiotherapy department for investigation or treatment. In the community, it might involve, for example, attending a healthcare appointment or going out with or visiting friends or family.

Decisions about implanted cardioverter-defibrillators

When a person who is approaching the end of their life has an implanted cardioverter-defibrillator (ICD), a discussion with them about CPR should also prompt a sensitive discussion about whether and when they may wish to have the shock function of their ICD deactivated if CPR attempts are not being recommended.

A proportion of people who die with an active ICD in place will receive shocks from the device in the last hours or days of their life. These are usually painful and can be distressing for the patient and for those close to them.

However, it must not be assumed that a recommendation not to attempt CPR automatically warrants deactivation of an ICD. Some people may wish to have prompt treatment from an ICD, but choose not to have CPR for cardiac arrest, which is much more traumatic, would have a lower chance of success and greater risk of harm.

Defining 'success' and 'futility' of CPR attempts

Achieving return of spontaneous circulation (ROSC) does not mean that CPR has been successful. A resuscitation attempt can only be regarded as successful if it restores a person to a duration and quality of life that they themselves regard as worth having.

Attempted resuscitation can only be regarded as being truly futile if it has no chance of achieving that outcome.

These statements emphasise the importance, whenever possible, of knowing a person's wishes, fears and beliefs in advance, and ideally documenting them in their own words. Achieving outcomes which are valuable to them, while avoiding those that are feared can be considered a success.

Predicting outcome

Predicting the outcome from CPR for cardiac arrest is far from easy. The outcome is dependent on many factors, including the prior state of health of the person and the times from arrest to starting CPR and attempting defibrillation as well as the time taken to achieve ROSC.

A scoring tool has been developed to predict chances of surviving attempted CPR with a good neurological outcome (Ebell et al.). Using this tool may assist in conversations with a person and those close to them, but it should not be used in isolation, since different people will value different outcomes.

Predictors of non-survival after attempted resuscitation have been published, but do not have sufficient predictive value to be used in general clinical practice in the immediate period after ROSC.

Avoiding discrimination

It is crucial that discussions and decisions are non-discriminatory and, for example, do not deprive people of CPR purely on the grounds of factors such as age or a disability.

The age of the person may be considered in the decision-making process but is only a relatively weak independent predictor of outcome. However, many elderly people have significant comorbidity, which influences outcome. Remember also to avoid discriminating by attempting CPR with no realistic chance of benefit on a person, simply because they are younger or because of an assumption that they would want this; opening discussions with people and those close to them can help prevent this.

Figure 5.3 A discussion around treatment and planning

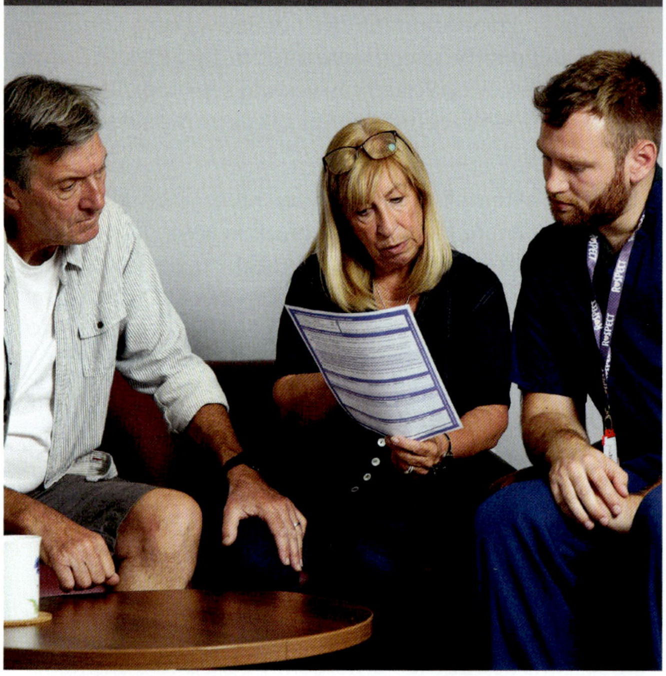

Decisions about CPR

If a decision whether or not to attempt CPR is taken at the moment of a cardiac arrest occurring.

The clinician must, as with all other clinical decisions made when a person lacks capacity, make a decision in that patient's holistic best interests, using whatever information they have available at that time. The presence of a completed emergency care and treatment plan can provide immediate guidance as to whether CPR should be initiated. Where a legally binding document exists, such as an appropriately completed advance decision to refuse CPR, then this must be adhered to if the circumstances given as to when this would be refused apply.

When to make a decision to attempt CPR

When finding someone in cardiac arrest, the default assumption should be to attempt CPR.

This allows time for those present to obtain sufficient information to determine the appropriateness of continuing resuscitation. This includes scenarios where there are recommendations not to attempt CPR in place, but the clinical situation is not that which was envisaged when the recommendation was recorded, for example, the cardiac arrest has been precipitated by a clearly reversible cause, such as choking, anaphylaxis, or an anaesthetic or intraoperative complication.

When to make a decision not to attempt CPR

1. CPR should never be attempted in those who have a legally binding document saying they do not want it. The legislation for this is different in the four nations and you should familiarise yourself with your local policy.
2. CPR should generally not be attempted in patients for whom a recorded recommendation not to attempt CPR has been made. These recommendations are made to ensure that people do not get treatments that are unlikely to work or outcomes they would not want. However, at the time of a cardiac arrest, the clinician must make a decision based on the current clinical situation and the information available to them. They should be satisfied that the circumstances of the arrest are those that were envisaged when the recommendation was recorded.
3. CPR should not be attempted where the death is clearly irreversible. Ambulance service guidelines allow appropriately trained clinicians to refrain from starting CPR in defined situations, for example in people with mortal injuries such as decapitation or hemicorporectomy, known submersion for more than 1.5 h, incineration, rigor mortis and hypostasis or where a person is known to be in the final stages of an advanced and irreversible condition, in which CPR would be both inappropriate and unsuccessful. In such cases, the ambulance clinician may recognise that death has occurred but cannot certify the cause of death (which in most countries can be done only by a doctor or Coroner).

   Similar recognition that death has occurred and is irreversible and a resulting decision not to start CPR may be made by doctors, experienced nurses or ambulance clinicians working in the community or in settings that provide care for people who are terminally or chronically ill. Whenever possible, advance recommendations about CPR should be considered as part of advance care planning before they are needed in a crisis.

Deciding to stop CPR

Many resuscitation attempts do not succeed in achieving ROSC and in those circumstances at some point, a decision has to be made to stop CPR. This decision can be made when continuing CPR will not achieve ROSC, or an outcome that would be valued by the person.

Factors influencing the decision will include the person's clinical history and prognosis, the cardiac arrest rhythm that is present, the response or absence of response to initial resuscitation measures, and the duration of the resuscitation attempt.

Do not discontinue resuscitation based on single criteria (e.g. pupil size, CPR duration, end-tidal carbon dioxide value, cardiac standstill on ultrasound, co-morbidities, lactate) as they are not sufficiently reliable in isolation to predict an adverse outcome.

Sometimes during a resuscitation attempt, information becomes available that was not known when CPR was started and indicates that CPR will not succeed or was not wanted. It is appropriate to stop CPR in those circumstances.

In general, CPR should be continued if a shockable rhythm or other potentially reversible cause for cardiac arrest persists. It is accepted that persistent asystole, in the absence of a reversible cause and with all Advanced Life Support (ALS) measures applied, is unlikely to be corrected by further CPR and is a reasonable basis for stopping a resuscitation attempt.

In some countries, including the UK, paramedics may cease a resuscitation attempt using similar criteria. Their strict protocol requires that conditions that might indicate a remote chance of survival (e.g. hypothermia) are absent, and the presence of asystole must also be established beyond reasonable doubt and documented on an ECG recording.

A decision to stop CPR should be made by the leader of the resuscitation attempt after consultation with other team members. Ultimately, the decision is based on a clinical judgement that further ALS is unlikely to restart the heart and breathing. When a decision is made to discontinue a resuscitation attempt, clear and accurate documentation of the events should be recorded including the rationale for stopping.

Special considerations

Certain circumstances at the time of cardiac arrest (e.g. hypothermia) enhance the chances of recovery without neurological damage. In such situations, do not use prognostic criteria (such as asystole persisting for a prolonged period); continue CPR until the reversible problem has been corrected (e.g. re-warming has been achieved).

Withdrawal of other treatment during the post-resuscitation period

It is difficult to predict the clinical and neurological outcome in people who remain unconscious during the first three days after ROSC. In general, other supportive treatment should be continued during this period, after which the prognosis can be assessed and predicted with greater confidence. This topic is covered in more detail in Chapter 13.

Auditing cardiac arrests, emergency care and treatment planning and decisions about CPR

Every cardiac arrest is best regarded as a critical clinical event, irrespective of the setting. The decisions made and actions taken by those present must be recorded clearly and accurately.

Local audit of such events should take place routinely, allowing recognition of good practice and corrective action to be undertaken where system failures have led to poor or absent decision-making, or inappropriate responses. Recording all arrests in one of the national databases (in-hospital: National Cardiac Arrest Audit, out-of-hospital: Out-of-hospital Cardiac Arrest Outcomes) will help to identify variation in practice and outcome to try to ensure equality of access to and delivery of treatment.

Health Service Circular 2000/028 states 'NHS Trust chief executives are asked to ensure that appropriate resuscitation policies which respect patients' rights are in place, understood by all relevant staff, and accessible to those who need them, and that such policies are subject to appropriate audit and monitoring arrangements.' As making anticipatory recommendations about emergency care and treatments, including CPR, is an integral part of good clinical care the decision-making process and the documentation of discussions and decisions about these should be audited routinely in all healthcare settings.

My key take-home messages from this chapter are:

05 SUMMARY LEARNING

Discussions and recommendations about CPR should be integrated into overarching emergency care and treatment plans such as ReSPECT.

Emergency care and treatment plans (including CPR) should be based on a careful assessment of each person's situation at any particular time. Do not apply blanket policies.

The patient (or those close to the patient if they lack capacity) must be consulted when making a recommendation not to attempt CPR.

Shared understanding and decision-making brings together the individual's expertise about themselves and what is important to them together with the clinician's knowledge about the benefits and risks of relevant treatments.

Establish a shared understanding of prognosis and treatments available, the patients values and fears and use these to agree on an overall treatment plan.

Situations where it is reasonable to not recommend attempting CPR include where it will not restart the heart and breathing for a sustained period, where the benefits of prolonging life outweigh the potential burdens and risks, or where the patient (or legal representative) refuses CPR.

Record recommendations clearly using terms that are understandable to those who may need to act on them. Avoid using terms which lack clarity on treatment goals.

In the event of cardiac arrest, CPR should be started unless a legally binding anticipatory decision has been made to not to attempt CPR, there are signs of irreversible death, or there is an applicable recommendation for CPR not to be attempted.

When there is a recommendation not to attempt CPR, CPR should generally not be attempted, unless the circumstances of the cardiac arrest are not those that which were anticipated when the recommendation was made (for example but not limited to choking, and intraoperative arrest)

Consider discontinuing CPR if it will not achieve ROSC or an outcome that would be valued by the person. Base decisions on a comprehensive assessment of relevant information. Do not rely on single criteria to predict outcome.

TEST YOURSELF QUESTIONS

1. What information should be documented in recording emergency care treatment plans?

Further reading

Becker C, Gross S, Beck K et al. A Randomized Trial of Shared Decision-Making in Code Status Discussions. NEJM Evidence. 2025 Apr 22;4(5)

British Medical Association, Resuscitation Council UK and Royal College of Nursing. Decisions relating to cardiopulmonary resuscitation. 3rd Edition, First revision 2016. www.resus.org.uk/library/publications/publication-decisions-relating-cardiopulmonary

Council of Europe. Guide on the decision-making process regarding medical treatment in end-of-life situations. http://www. coe.int/en/web/portal/-/council-of-europe-launches-a-guide-on- the-decision-making-process- regarding-medical-treatment-in- end-of-life-situations

Ebell MH, Jang W, Shen Y, Geocadin RG; Get With the Guidelines–Resuscitation Investigators. Development and validation of the Good Outcome Following Attempted Resuscitation (GO-FAR) score to predict neurologically intact survival after in-hospital cardiopulmonary resuscitation. JAMA Intern Med. 2013 Nov 11;173(20):1872-8. doi: 10.1001/jamainternmed.2013.10037. Erratum in: JAMA Intern Med. 2015 Jul;175(7):1247-8. doi: 10.1001/jamainternmed.2015.2890. PMID: 24018585

Fritz Z, Slowther AM, Perkins G. Resuscitation policy should focus on the patient, not the decision. BMJ 2017;356:j813.

General Medical Council. Treatment and care towards the end of life: good practice in decision-making. 2010. www.gmc-uk.org

Hawkes CA, Fritz Z, Deas G, et al. Development of the Recommended Summary Plan for eEmergency Care and Treatment (ReSPECT). Resuscitation. 2020;148:98-107.

Meek T, Clyburn R, Fritz Z, Pitcher D, Ruck Keene A, Young PJ. Implementing advance care plans in the peri-operative period, including plans for cardiopulmonary resuscitation: Association of Anaesthetists clinical practice guideline. Anaesthesia. 2022 Apr; 77(4):456-462

Mentzelopoulos S, Couper K, Van De Voorde P et al. European Resuscitation Council Guidelines for Resuscitation 2021 Ethics of Resuscitation and End-of-Life Decisions. Resuscitation 2021 In press.

Perkins GD, Griffiths F, Slowther AM, et al. Do-not-attempt-cardiopulmonary-resuscitation decisions: an evidence synthesis. NIHR Journals Library; 2016 Apr. https://www.journalslibrary.nihr. ac.uk/hsdr/hsdr04110/#/abstract

Perkins GD, Hawkes C, Eli et al. Evaluation of the Recommended Summary Plan for Emergency Care and Treatment. NIHR Journals Library; 2021 https://www.journalslibrary.nihr.ac.uk/programmes/ hsdr/151509/#/

Pitcher D, Soar J, Hogg K, et al: the CIED Working Group. Cardiovascular implanted electronic devices in people towards the end of life, during cardiopulmonary resuscitation and after death: guidance from the Resuscitation Council (UK), British Cardiovascular Society and National Council for Palliative Care. Heart 2016;102:A1-A17.

Pitcher D, Fritz Z, Wang M, Spiller, J. Emergency care and resuscitation plans. BMJ 2017;356:j876.

R (Tracey) v Cambridge University Hospitals NHS Foundation Trust & Ors EWHC 3670 (Admin). 2014. https://www.judiciary.uk/wp-content/uploads/2014/06/tracey-approved.pdf

Raffay V, Lauridsen KG, Wittig J, et al. European Resuscitation Council Guidelines 2025: Ethics in Resuscitation. Resuscitation. 2025. In print.

Resuscitation Council UK. British Cardiovascular Society and National Council for Palliative Care. Deactivation of implantable cardioverter-defibrillators towards the end of life. www.resus.org.uk

Resuscitation Council UK. CPR, AEDs and the law. https://www.resus.org.uk/library/publications/publication-cpr-aeds-and-law

The Scottish Government. Adults with Incapacity (Scotland) Act 2000: A short guide to the Act. www.gov.scot/Topics/Justice/law/ awi/010408awiwebpubs/infopublications

UK Government. Mental Capacity Act 2005 Code of Practice. Mental Capacity Act Code of Practice – GOV.UK (www.gov.uk)

Winspear v City Hospitals Sunderland NHSFT EWHC 3250 (QB), QB 691. 2015. https://www.bailii.org/ew/cases/EWHC/QB/2015/3250.html

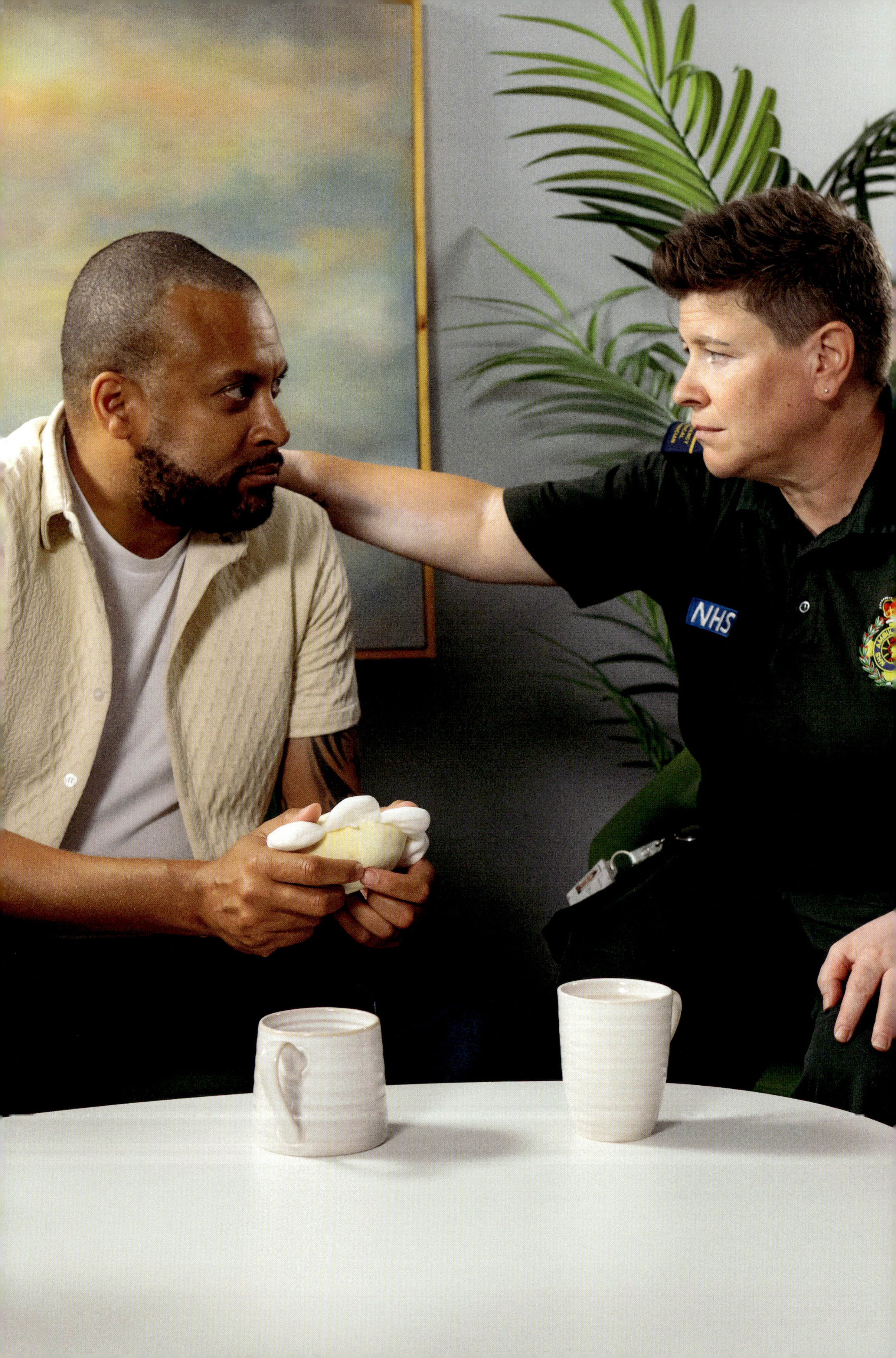
NHS

06 Supporting relatives and responders in resuscitation practice

In this chapter

The involvement of relatives and friends

Caring for the recently bereaved

Responder wellbeing

The learning outcomes will enable you to:

Know how to support relatives witnessing attempted resuscitation

Know how to care for the recently bereaved

Consider the religious and cultural requirements when a patient has died

Consider the legal and practical arrangements following a recent death

Support team members

Throughout this chapter, the term 'relatives' includes close friends, family, and other people important to the patient.

Introduction

In many cases of out-of-hospital cardiac arrest, the person who performs CPR will be a close friend or relative, and they may wish to remain with the patient. Many relatives find it more distressing to be separated from their family member during these critical moments than to witness attempts at resuscitation.

Healthcare professionals should consider the preferences of patients and their relatives.

If the resuscitation attempt fails, relatives perceive several advantages of being present during resuscitation:

- It helps them come to terms with the reality of death, reducing the severity or duration of grief.
- The relative can speak while there is still a chance that the dying person can hear.
- They are not distressed by being separated from a loved one at a time when they feel the need to be present.
- They can see that everything possible was done for the dying person, which helps with their understanding of the reality of the situation.
- They can touch and speak with the deceased while the body is warm.

There are also potential disadvantages to relatives being present:

- The resuscitation attempt may be distressing, particularly if the relatives are not kept informed.
- Relatives may physically or emotionally hinder the staff involved in the resuscitation attempt. Actions or remarks by medical or nursing staff may offend grieving family members.
- Relatives may be disturbed by the memory of events, although evidence indicates that fantasy (about unwitnessed events) is worse than fact (about events that have been seen). Staff should consider the expectations of the bereaved and their cultural background during and after the death.
- Relatives may demonstrate their emotions vocally or physically, whilst others may wish to sit quietly or read religious text. The staff must have sufficient insight, knowledge and skills to anticipate individual needs and identify potential problems.

The involvement of relatives and friends

Care and consideration of relatives during resuscitation becomes increasingly important as procedures become more invasive.

Support should be provided by an appropriately qualified healthcare professional whose responsibility is to care for family members witnessing cardiopulmonary resuscitation. This member of staff should ideally not be undertaking clinical duties during the resuscitation attempt.

Figure 6.1 Taking over from the first responder

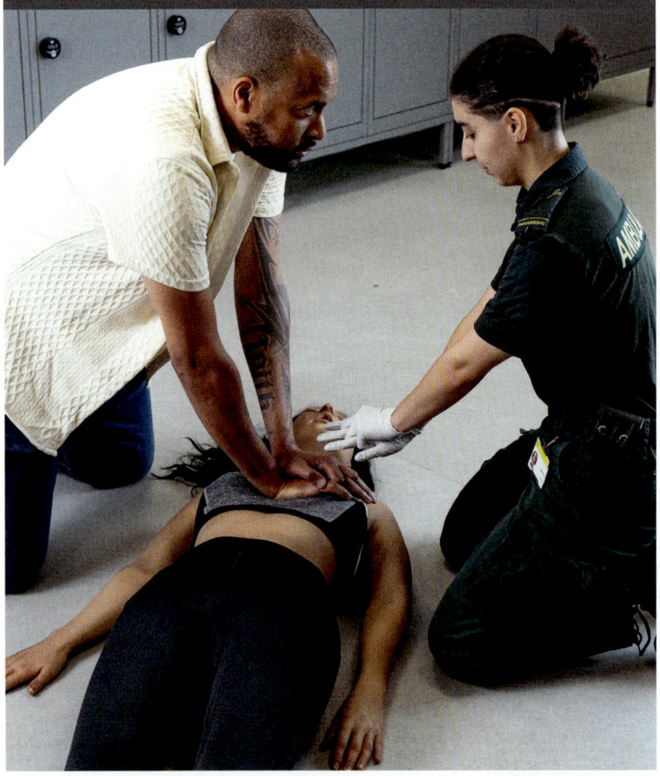

Figure 6.2 Support being provided by an appropriately qualified healthcare professional

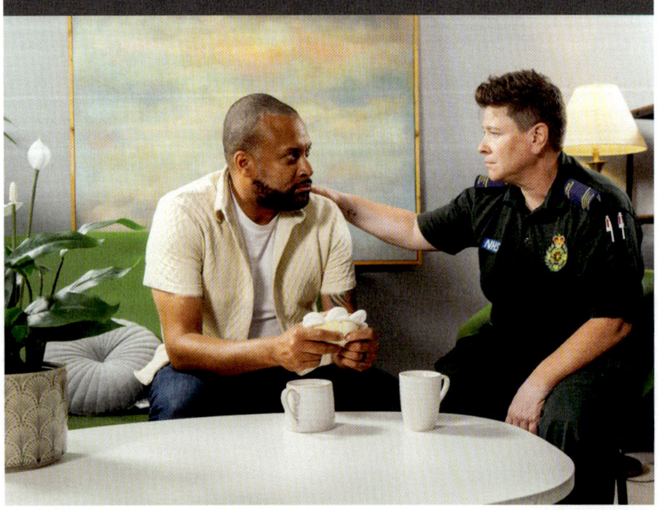

The identified member of staff should adopt the following safeguards:

Where possible, resuscitation teams should allow relatives the opportunity to observe the attempted resuscitation of their loved one.

Acknowledge the difficulty of the situation.
Ensure that they understand they have a choice about whether to be present during resuscitation.
Avoid provoking feelings of guilt, whatever their decision is.

Explain that they will be looked after whether or not they decide to witness the resuscitation attempt.
Ensure that introductions are made and names are known.

Ensure that relatives understand that they will be able to leave and return at any time and will always be accompanied.

Give a clear explanation of what has happened in terms of the illness or injury and what they can expect to see when they enter the resuscitation area.

Ask relatives not to interfere with the resuscitation process, but offer them the opportunity to touch the patient when they are told that it is safe to do so.

Explain the nature of procedures in simple terms.
If resuscitation is unsuccessful, explain why the attempt has been stopped.

If the patient dies, advise the relatives that there may be a brief interval while equipment is removed, after which they can return to be together in private.

Offer the relatives time to think about what has happened and the opportunity for further questions.

Caring for the recently bereaved

Caring for the bereaved compassionately will ease the grieving process. Adapt the following considerations to the individual relatives and their cultural needs:

- Early contact with one person, usually an experienced healthcare professional.
- Provision of a suitable area for relatives to wait (e.g. relatives' room).
- Break bad news sympathetically and support the grief response appropriately.
- Arrange for relatives to view the body.
- Religious and pastoral care requirements.
- Legal and practical arrangements.
- Follow up and team support.

Early contact with one person

Ideally, this should be the person who has supported the relatives during the resuscitation attempt.

If the resuscitation attempt was not observed, allocate a member of the care team specifically to support the relatives. Communication between the emergency services and the receiving hospital should ensure that the arrival of relatives is anticipated for an out-of-hospital arrest. A warm, friendly and confident greeting will help to establish an open and honest relationship.

Provision of a suitable room

This should provide the appropriate ambience, space and privacy for relatives to ask questions and to express their emotions freely.

Table 6.1 SPIKES model for breaking bad news

S	Setting up	Establish an appropriate setting.
P	Perception	Check the patient or relative's perception of the situation prompting the news regarding the illness or test results.
I	Invitation	Determine the amount of information known or how much information is desired.
K	Knowledge	Know the medical facts and their implication before initiating the conversation.
E	Emotions with empathy	Explore the emotions raised during the conversation and respond with empathy.
S	Summary	Summarise and establish a strategy for support.

Breaking bad news and supporting the grief response

An uncomplicated and honest approach will help avoid mixed messages. The most appropriate person should be the one to break the bad news to the relatives. It may be more appropriate for the healthcare professional who has been accompanying the relatives to break the news. However, relatives may also find comfort in speaking with the most senior clinician present, and this opportunity should always be offered.

SPIKES Model for Breaking Bad News provides a practical step-wise framework for communication (Table 6.1).

Other considerations include:

- Confirm that you are talking with the correct relatives and establish their relationship to the deceased. Briefly establish what they know and use this as the basis for your communication with them.
- Use tone of voice and non-verbal behaviour to support what you are saying. Use simple words and avoid medical jargon and platitudes that will be meaningless to relatives. Use the word 'dead', 'died' or 'death' so that there is no ambiguity.
- When breaking bad news, allow periods of silence for relatives to absorb and think about what they have been told.
- Anticipate the different types of reaction/emotional response you may experience after breaking bad news. Possible responses to grief include acute emotional distress/shock, anger, denial/disbelief, guilt and catatonia.
- An individual's gender, age, cultural background and lived experience may influence the response to grief. Respect cultural requirements and, where possible, provide written support where needed.

Arrange viewing of the body

Many newly bereaved relatives value the opportunity to view their loved ones. Their experience is likely to be affected by whether the deceased appears in a presentable condition. Advise relatives what to expect before they view the body, particularly if the deceased has suffered any mutilating injuries. People are less concerned about medical devices and equipment than is generally believed. Being in the physical presence of their loved one will help them work through the grieving process. Ensure the opportunity to touch or hold the deceased is given. Staff should accompany relatives during the viewing process and remain nearby to offer support or provide information as needed.

Religious requirements, legal and practical arrangements

A patient's religious convictions influence variations in handling the body and expressions of grief.

The resuscitation team should take into account the patient's and their relatives' beliefs, values, and cultural and religious rituals. There is an increasing emphasis on the need for care practice to be culturally sensitive, as a way of valuing and respecting the cultural and religious needs of patients. Religious representatives from the patient's denomination or faith are usually available to attend in-hospital. Hospital chaplains and spiritual care teams are a valuable source of strength and information for families and staff. Prayers, blessings, and religious acts and procedures are all important in ensuring that relatives are not further distressed. It is also important to respect the views and wishes of those who are not religious.

Legal and practical arrangements following death are equally important. These include:

- Notification of the coroner or other appropriate authority.
- Notification of the patient's family doctor.
- Organ and tissue donation decisions.
- Provision of information about what to do after a relative's death.
- Adherence to hospital procedure regarding the return of patients' property and valuables.
- Information concerning social services that are available.
- Information concerning post-mortem examination, where indicated.
- Follow-up arrangements for relatives, which may involve long-term counselling.
- Provision of a telephone contact number for relatives to use and a named staff member whom they can call should they have any further questions.

Supporting responders

Unfortunately, the likelihood of death for patients sustaining cardiac arrest is high, despite efforts to resuscitate them. Resuscitation exposure can evoke a range of emotions, from positive to neutral to negative.

Distress is common, and there are also mental health conditions commonly associated with resuscitation exposure, such as post-traumatic stress disorder (PTSD), depression, and anxiety.

Suicidal thoughts are surprisingly common, and people do not have to be depressed to be suicidal. Knowledge of these conditions can help to anticipate and recognise potential development of mental health conditions (Table 6.2).

Remember that responders can include members of the public or the patient's relatives (particularly at out-of-hospital cardiac arrests) as well as healthcare professionals.

RCUK have a dedicated webpage to support those affected by cardiac arrest, available at www.resus.org.uk/public-resource/support-after-cardiac-arrest

SCAN ME
for support after
cardiac arrest

Table 6.2 Acute stress reactions adapted from Walton, Murray and Christian 2020

Physical	Behavioural	Emotional	Cognitive
Palpitations	Avoidance	Numbness	Poor concentration
Nausea, low appetite	Recklessness	Anxiety	Intrusive thoughts
Chest pain	Detachment	Low mood	Flashbacks
Headaches	Withdrawal	Anger, fear	Poor memory
Abdominal pains	Irritability	Mood swings	Confusion
Insomnia	Drug or alcohol abuse	Loss of pleasure	Hyper vigilance
Hyper arousal	Conflicts with others	Low confidence	Rumination

Figure 6.3 Post-resuscitation procedure

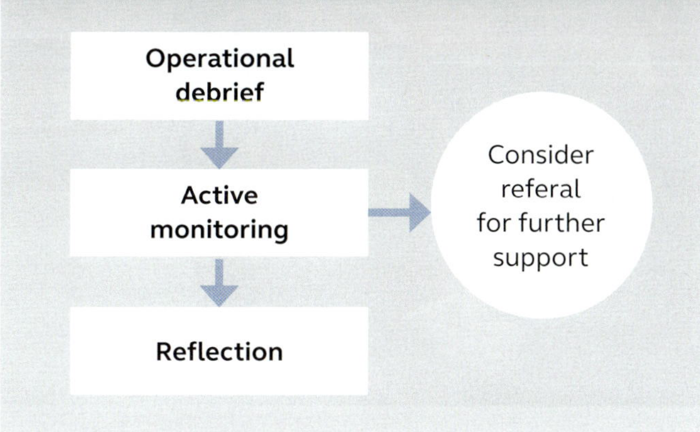

Figure 6.4 STOP-5 – an example of a structured framework for debriefing

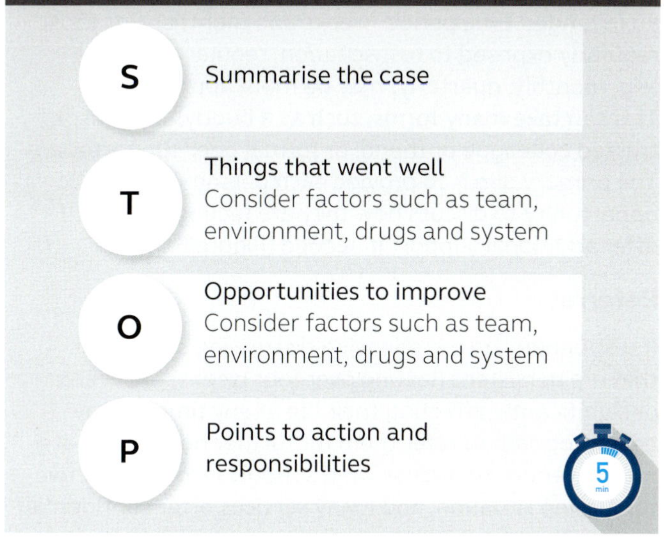

Post-resuscitation procedure

A 'post-resuscitation procedure' (Figure 6.3) is suggested for responders to follow after resuscitation exposure. The key aim is to identify and support people who are negatively impacted as early as possible.

Operational debriefing (OD)

An OD is led by the clinical team and is a learning conversation that primarily focuses on the team's performance. In other words, how can lessons be learned from this event and improve the performance next time?

OD is recommended to improve patient outcomes, particularly when data-driven approaches are employed. This means, for example, using defibrillator impedance signal recording to measure the effectiveness of CPR or video footage to assess resuscitation objectively. When using patient identifiable data, ensure that all relevant patient privacy and medico-legal requirements have been met.

The OD can be done individually or as a group. ODs can be undertaken immediately after the resuscitation or in the following days or weeks. There are many methods of OD and a lot of variation between organisations. For example, a model like STOP5 may be used (Figure 6.4).

To perform the STOP 5 debrief, first gather the team for five minutes, then:

- Summarise the case (create a shared narrative of what happened).
- Things that went well (ask the team)
- Opportunities to improve (ask the team).
- Points of action and who will be responsible, e.g.:
  - Which equipment will be restocked and by whom?
  - Should and how will we share what we have learnt?
  - A team member is distressed. Who will check on them?
  - Is a time-out required?

The OD is also an opportunity to support responders in the following ways:

- Reassure responders that their immediate reactions & feelings are common to reduce stigma.
- Educate on possible (negative) reactions in the coming days, weeks or months and reassure that these usually reduce over time. Signpost when (if reactions are persistent, severe or affecting life) and where (with a trusted friend, Supervisor, Occupational Health, GP, Mental Health charities) to seek further support.
- Offer a break from the shift to reset.
- Assign a 'buddy' to check in on each other or take contact details for active monitoring.
- Check the understanding of performance limits and futility to avoid a responder overestimating their personal influence over a poor outcome and leaving a resuscitation believing (usually incorrectly) 'if only I did that differently, they would have lived'.

Note that 1:1 psychologically focused debriefing is not recommended, and there is no role for mental health professionals to be 'flown in' to provide immediate psychological assistance to responders who have been involved in a resuscitation. There is little evidence for ODs formally preventing the onset of mental health conditions; however, responders report feeling more supported after ODs, and evidence available indicates that well-conducted ODs are unlikely to cause psychological harm.

Therefore, while the OD is primarily a learning and performance improvement tool, it is an opportunity to support responder wellbeing as part of the post-resuscitation procedure. All team members are encouraged to participate in an OD, but it should not be mandatory. Anything discussed in the OD should be treated as confidential.

Active monitoring

Create opportunities to 'check in' with responders over an extended time period (weeks and months). For those regularly exposed to resuscitation, regular check-ins (e.g. monthly, quarterly) may be more appropriate. This can take many forms, such as a buddy, supervisor, trusted colleague or friend, or formal peer supporters. The primary aim is to provide each person with the opportunity to discuss how they are feeling and to offer additional support if needed (Figure 6.5).

Referral

If responders are experiencing distressing symptoms that are persistent (lasting over four weeks) or severe, or significantly affecting their life at any time, it may be appropriate to refer them for further help. There are many avenues to discuss what support is most effective for a given situation, and many services offer confidential advice if in doubt. Some people may not wish to be referred to services, and it is important to respect their wishes, provided they are not at risk of immediate harm to themselves or others. It is usually a good idea to inform a supervisor or a trusted colleague at work about the situation so they can assist with active monitoring, developing a recovery plan, and providing further support if needed.

Figure 6.5 Checking in with a colleague

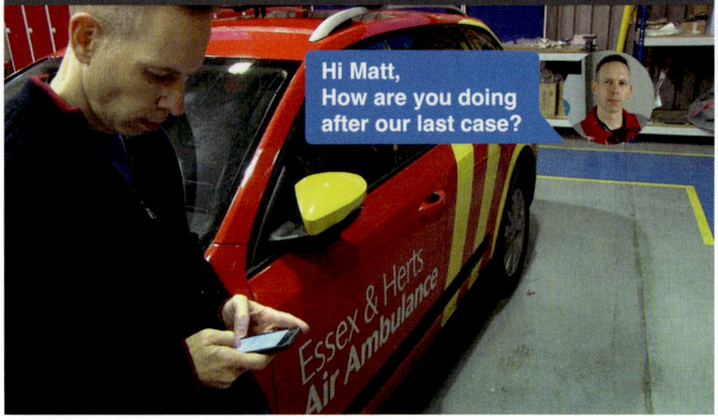
Hi Matt,
How are you doing
after our last case?
Essex & Herts
Air Ambulance

Reflection

Periodic team reflection sessions help to share experiences that may otherwise go unspoken and process emotional challenges together. Ideally, this can be led by a supervisor and is not necessarily tied to a single event. This also creates an opportunity to check in with and support each other.

06 SUMMARY LEARNING

Many relatives want the opportunity to be present during the attempted resuscitation of their loved one. This may help the grieving process.

Communication with relatives during resuscitation and after bereavement should be honest, straightforward, and supportive.

Responders can develop distress and mental health conditions because of resuscitation exposure and their working environment.

Post-resuscitation procedure supports responders and facilitates early access to help if required.

Debriefing is a learning conversation designed to improve subsequent performance. It is also an opportunity to support responder wellbeing as part of the post-resuscitation procedure.

There are many factors influencing responder Wellbeing, and there are opportunities to support Responder Wellbeing at every level.

Further reading

Jabre P, Tazarourte K, Azoulay E, et al. Offering the opportunity for family to be present during cardiopulmonary resuscitation: 1-year assessment. Intensive Care Med 2014;40:981–7.

Office for National Statistics Death certification advisory group September 2018, Guidance for Doctors completing medical certificates of cause of death in England & Wales.

Porter J, Cooper S, Sellick K. Attitudes, implementation and practice of family presence during Resuscitation (FPDR): A qualitative literature review. International Emergency Nursing 2013;21:26-34.

Scottish Government, What To Do After A Death In Scotland - Practical Advice For Times Of Bereavement - 11th edition Scottish Government 16 Nov 2016.

Watts, J Death, Dying and Bereavement: Issues for practice. Dunedin 2010.

Baile WF, Buckman R, Lenzi R, Glober G, Beale EA, Kudelka AP. SPIKES—a six-step protocol for delivering bad news: application to the patient with cancer. Oncologist. 2000;5(1):302–311.

Walker C. "STOP 5: stop for 5 minutes" – our bespoke hot debrief model. 2018 https://www.edinburghemergencymedicine.com/ blog/2018/11/1/stop-5-stop-for-5-minutes-our-bespoke-hot- debrief-model.

Spencer SA, Nolan JP, Osborn M, Georgiou A. The presence of psychological trauma symptoms in resuscitation providers and an exploration of debriefing practices. Resuscitation. 2019 Sep;142:175-181.

Resuscitation Council UK, Support after cardiac arrest, https://www.resus.org.uk/public-resource/support-after-cardiac-arrest

Resuscitation Council UK, Responder Wellbeing. https://www.resus.org.uk/responder-wellbeing

My key take-home messages from this chapter are:

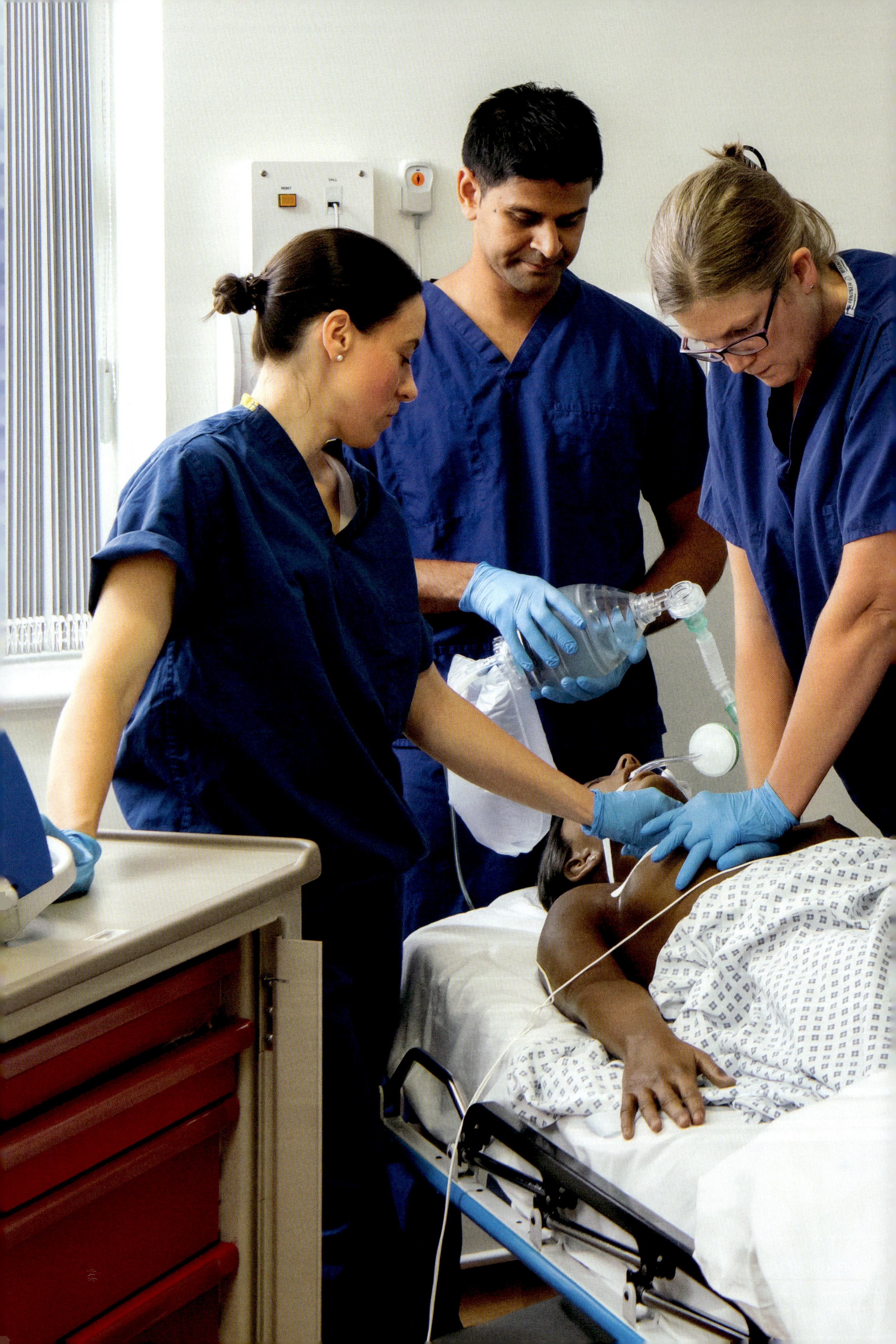

07 Advanced Life Support algorithm

In this chapter

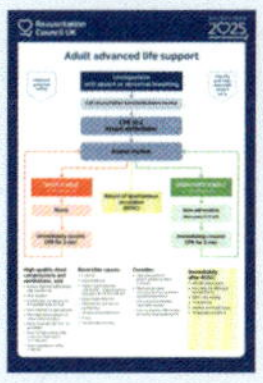

The adult advanced life support (ALS) algorithm

Shockable and non-shockable rhythms

The learning outcomes will enable you to:

Follow the ALS algorithm

Understand the importance of minimally interrupted high-quality chest compressions

Identify and treat relevant shockable and non-shockable rhythms

Consider potentially reversible causes of cardiac arrest

Introduction

Heart rhythms associated with cardiac arrest are divided into two groups:

- **Shockable rhythms (ventricular fibrillation/pulseless ventricular tachycardia (VF/pVT)).**
- **Non-shockable rhythms (asystole and pulseless electrical activity (PEA)).**

The main difference in the treatment of these two groups of arrhythmias is the need for defibrillation in patients with VF/pVT. Other actions, common to both groups, include chest compressions, airway management and ventilation, venous access, injection of medication and the identification and correction of reversible causes.

The ALS algorithm (Figure 7.1) is a standardised approach for patients in cardiac arrest.

The ALS algorithm has the advantage of enabling treatment to be delivered expediently, without protracted discussion.

Each member of the resuscitation team can predict and prepare for the next stage in the patient's treatment, making the team more efficient.

The most important interventions that improve survival after cardiac arrest are early and uninterrupted high-quality chest compressions and early defibrillation for VF/pVT.

Although drugs and advanced airways are still included among ALS interventions, they are of secondary importance to high-quality, uninterrupted chest compressions and early defibrillation.

Chapter 8 deals with the recognition of cardiac arrest rhythms. If you are not experienced or trained in recognising cardiac arrest rhythms, use an automated external defibrillator (AED). Some defibrillators have both a manual and AED capability. Once switched on, the AED will give voice and visual prompts that will guide you through the correct sequence of actions.

Figure 7.2 Ventricular fibrillation

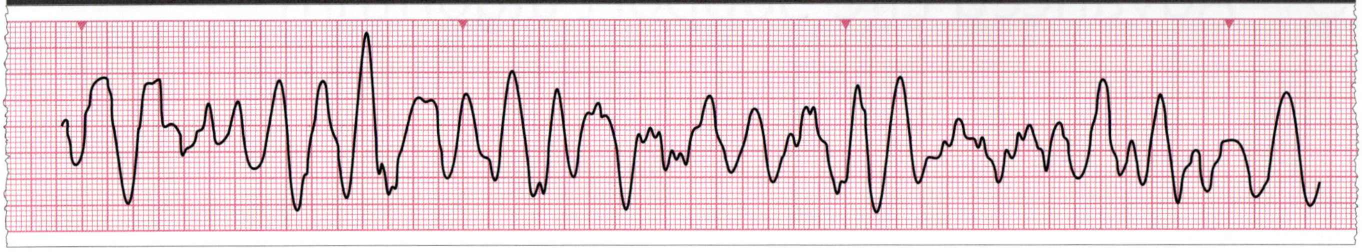

Shockable rhythms (VF/pVT)

In approximately 20% of all cardiac arrests, the initial presenting rhythm will be VF or pVT (Figure 7.2).

Treatment of shockable rhythms (VF/pVT)

A manual defibrillator is used in the sequence described below. Further information about defibrillation can be found in Chapter 3.

1. **Confirm cardiac arrest –** check for normal breathing and signs of life. If trained to do so, simultaneously check for a central pulse for less than 10 seconds.
2. **If there are no signs of life,** call for the resuscitation team.
3. **Commence uninterrupted chest compressions** while applying self-adhesive defibrillation pads. Ensure that the apical (lateral) pad is positioned correctly (i.e. directly below the armpit in the mid-axillary line).
4. **Plan actions** before pausing CPR for rhythm analysis and communicate these to the team.
5. **Briefly pause chest compressions** (less than 5 seconds) to confirm the rhythm is shockable (VF/pVT).
6. **Resume chest compressions immediately;** warn all rescuers other than the individual performing chest compressions to "stand clear" and remove any oxygen delivery device as appropriate.
7. **The team member** responsible for defibrillation should select the appropriate energy level and charge the defibrillator (Figure 7.3). Choose an energy setting of at least 150 J for the first shock, the same or a higher energy for subsequent shocks, or follow the manufacturer's guidance for the particular defibrillator being used.
8. **Ensure that the rescuer giving the compressions is the only person touching the patient.**
9. **Once the defibrillator is charged and the safety check is complete,** instruct the rescuer performing chest compressions to "stand clear." When clear, administer the shock (Figure 7.4).
10. **After shock delivery, immediately restart CPR** (Figure 7.5), starting with chest compressions. **Do not** pause to reassess the rhythm or feel for a pulse. The pause in chest compressions is to enable safe shock delivery and should be very brief, lasting no longer than 5 seconds.
11. **Continue CPR for 2 minutes;** the team leader prepares the team for the next pause in CPR.
12. **Briefly pause at the end of the 2-minute cycle** to re-analyse the heart rhythm.
13. **If VF/pVT, repeat steps 6–12 above** and deliver a second shock.
14. **If VF/pVT persists, repeat steps 6–9 above** and deliver a third shock. Resume chest compressions immediately. Give adrenaline 1 mg IV/IO and amiodarone 300 mg IV/IO while performing a further 2-minute cycle. Withhold adrenaline if there are signs of return of spontaneous circulation (ROSC) during CPR.
15. **After three shocks, consider using a defibrillation vector change** by using an alternative defibrillation pad position (e.g. antero-posterior). Prepare to place a fresh set of pads with minimal interruptions in chest compressions.
16. **Repeat this 2-minute CPR** – rhythm/pulse check – defibrillation sequence if VF/pVT persists.
17. **Give further adrenaline 1 mg IV after alternate cycles** (i.e. approximately every 3–5 minutes).
18. **If organised electrical activity compatible with a cardiac output is seen during a rhythm check**, seek evidence of return of spontaneous circulation (ROSC) (check for signs of life, a central pulse, and end-tidal carbon dioxide ($ETCO_2$) on waveform capnography if available):
    a. If there is ROSC, start post-resuscitation care.
    b. If there are no signs of ROSC, and there is organised electrical activity, this is PEA and switch to the non-shockable side of the algorithm.
19. **If asystole is seen,** continue CPR and switch to the non-shockable side of the algorithm.

Adult advanced life support

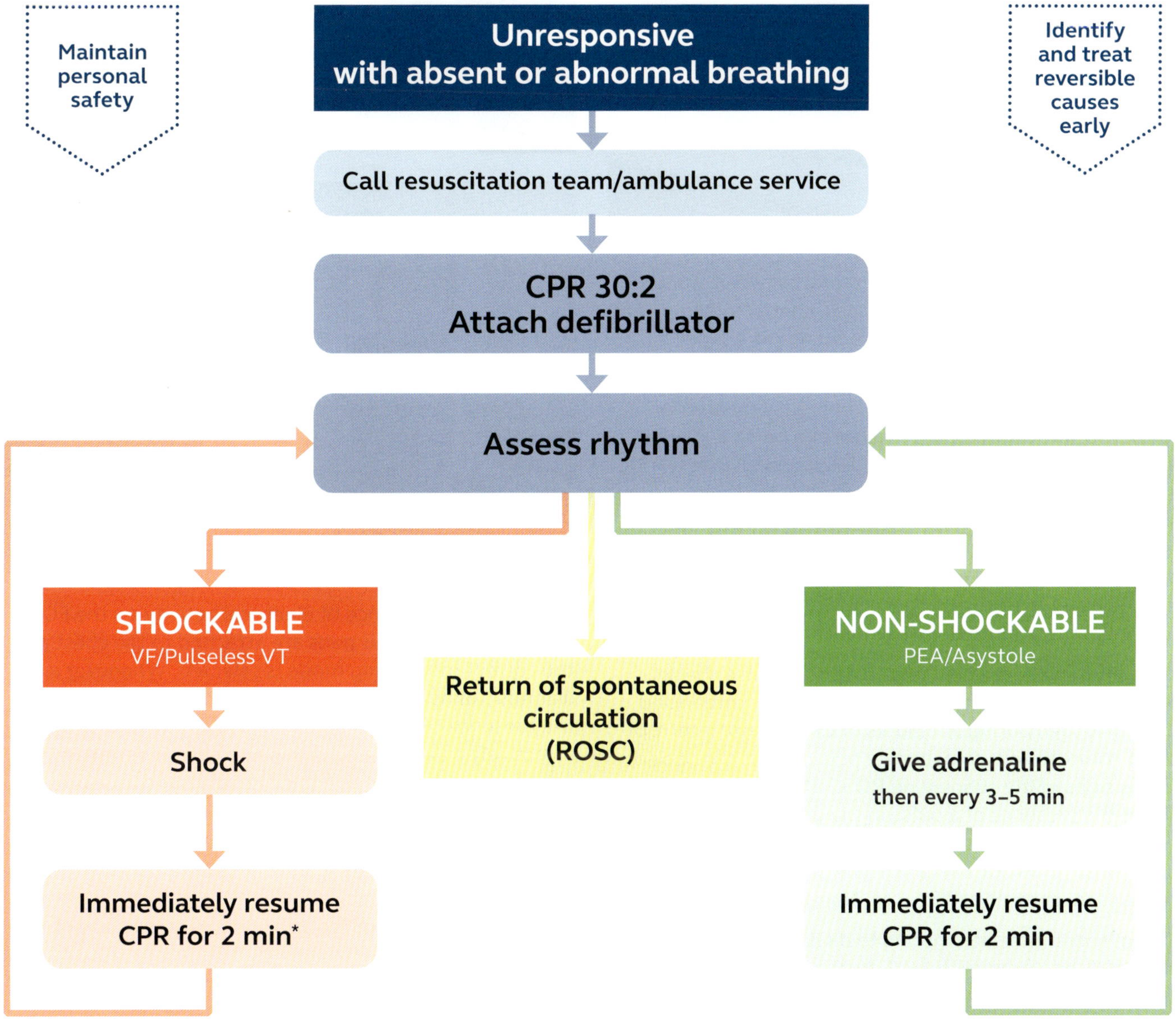

High-quality chest compressions and ventilations, and:

- Ensure optimal defibrillator pad placement
- Give oxygen
- Continuous compressions if tracheal tube or SGA
- Use waveform capnography
- Minimise interruptions to chest compressions
- Early IV access (IO if IV not possible)

* Give 1st adrenaline after 3 shocks, then every 3–5 minutes

* Give amiodarone after 3 shocks

Reversible causes:

- Hypoxia
- Hypovolaemia
- Hyper-hypokalaemia, -calcaemia, -magnesaemia, hypoglycaemia (metabolic)
- Hypo-hyperthermia
- Thrombosis (coronary/ pulmonary)
- Tension pneumothorax
- Toxins
- Tamponade (cardiac)

Consider:

- Changing pads to antero-posterior after 3 shocks
- Mechanical chest compressions to facilitate transfer/treatment
- Ultrasound to identify reversible causes
- Extracorporeal CPR and/or coronary angiography/PCI

Immediately after ROSC:

- ABCDE assessment
- Aim SpO_2 94–98% and normal $PaCO_2$
- SBP > 100 mmHg
- 12-lead ECG
- Identify and treat cause
- Temperature control

Figure 7.1 Adult advanced life support (ALS) algorithm

Figure 7.3 Continue chest compressions during defibrillator charging – everyone else stands clear

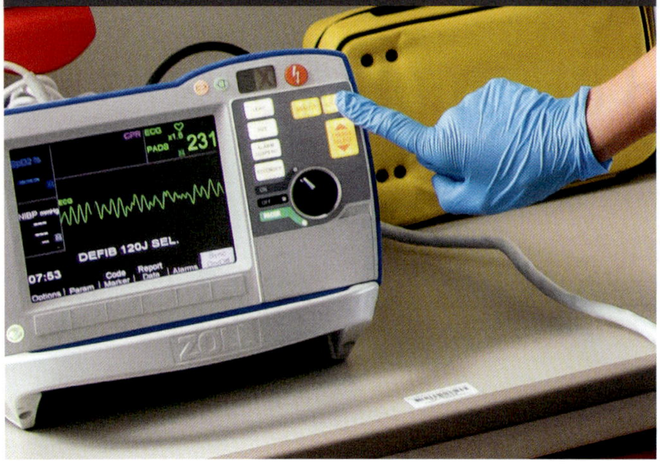

It is important to minimise the interval between stopping compressions and delivering a shock. Longer interruptions to chest compressions reduce the chance of a shock restoring a spontaneous circulation.

Chest compressions are resumed immediately after a shock without checking the rhythm or a pulse because even if the defibrillation attempt is successful in restoring a perfusing rhythm, it is very rare for a pulse to be palpable immediately after defibrillation and the delay in trying to palpate a pulse will further compromise the myocardium if a perfusing rhythm has not been restored. If a perfusing rhythm has been restored, giving chest compressions does not increase the chance of VF recurring.

Keep rhythm checks brief and undertake pulse checks only if an organised rhythm is observed. If an organised rhythm is seen during 2 minutes of CPR, do not interrupt chest compressions to palpate a pulse unless the patient shows signs of life suggesting ROSC. If there is any doubt about the presence of a pulse in the presence of an organised rhythm, resume CPR. If the patient has ROSC, begin post-resuscitation care. If the patient's rhythm changes to asystole or PEA, see 'Non-shockable rhythms'.

Do not spend time attempting to distinguish fine VF from coarse VF, or extremely fine VF from asystole. If the rhythm appears to be VF, give a shock, and if it appears to be asystole, continue chest compressions. Avoid excessive interruptions in chest compression for rhythm analysis. Rescuers who are not comfortable with rapid rhythm assessment during CPR should use an automated external defibrillator.

Non-shockable rhythms (PEA and asystole)

Pulseless electrical activity (PEA) is defined as a cardiac arrest in the presence of electrical activity that would normally be associated with a palpable pulse. These patients often have some mechanical myocardial contractions, but they are too weak to produce a detectable pulse or blood pressure. PEA may be caused by reversible conditions that can be treated (see below). Survival following cardiac arrest with asystole or PEA is unlikely unless a reversible cause can be found and treated quickly and effectively.

Figure 7.4 Stand clear – no-one touches the patient when the shock is delivered

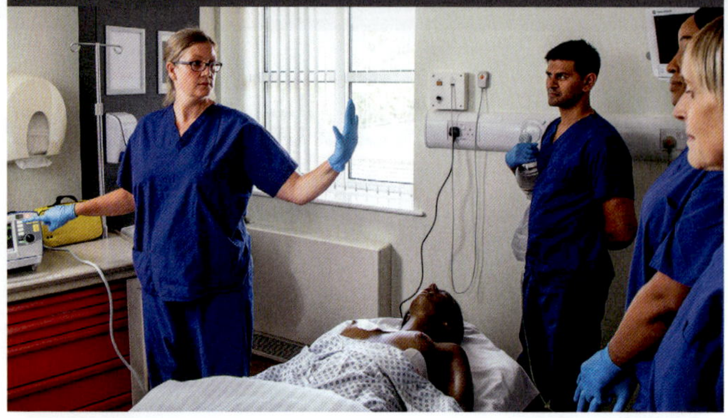

Figure 7.5 Restart chest compressions immediately after shock delivery

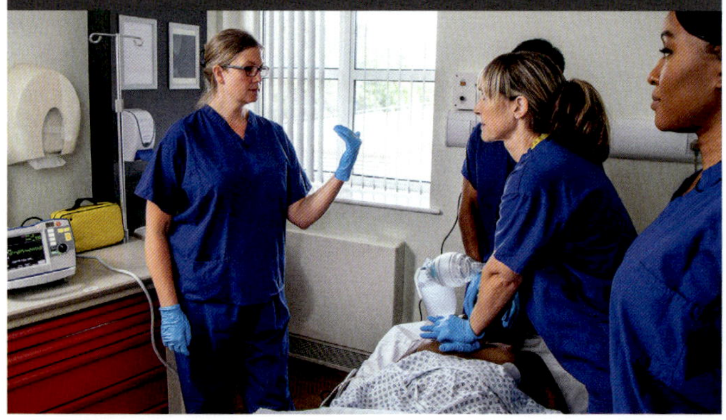

Asystole is the absence of electrical activity on the ECG trace. Ensure the ECG pads are attached to the chest and the correct monitoring mode is selected. Whenever a diagnosis of asystole is made, carefully check the ECG for the presence of P waves, as ventricular standstill may be effectively treated by cardiac pacing in this situation. Attempts to pace true asystole are unlikely to be successful.

Treatment for non-shockable rhythms (PEA and asystole)

1. Check for signs of life and confirm cardiac arrest.
2. Call the resuscitation team.
3. Commence uninterrupted chest compressions while applying self-adhesive defibrillation pads. Ensure that the apical (lateral) pad is positioned correctly (i.e. directly below the armpit in the mid-axillary line).
4. Plan actions before pausing CPR for rhythm analysis and communicate these to the team.
5. Briefly pause chest compressions (less than 5 seconds) to confirm the rhythm is non-shockable.
6. Administer 1 mg of adrenaline IV as soon as intravascular access is established.
7. Continue CPR when the patient has an advanced airway in place, deliver continuous chest compressions without pausing for ventilations, which should be delivered at a rate of 10 breaths min^{-1}.

8. Recheck the rhythm at the end of the 2-minute cycle.
9. If electrical activity compatible with a pulse is seen, check for a pulse and/or signs of life.
10. If a pulse and/or signs of life are present, start post-resuscitation care.
11. If no pulse and/or no signs of life are present (PEA or asystole):
    a. Continue CPR.
    b. Recheck the rhythm after 2 min and proceed accordingly.
    c. Give further adrenaline 1 mg IV every 3–5 min. Once adrenaline has been administered, it should be given every 3–5 min regardless of which side of the algorithm you are following.

- If VF/pVT is seen at rhythm check, change to the shockable side of the algorithm.

During CPR

During cardiac arrest, emphasis is placed on high-quality chest compressions between defibrillation attempts, recognising and treating reversible causes (Four Hs and Four Ts), obtaining a secure airway, and vascular access.

During CPR with a compression to ventilation ratio of 30:2, the underlying rhythm may be seen clearly on the monitor during the pauses for ventilation. If VF/pVT is seen during this brief pause (whether on the shockable or non-shockable side of the algorithm), do not attempt defibrillation at this stage; instead, continue with CPR until the 2-minute cycle is completed. Knowing that the rhythm is VF/pVT, the team should be fully prepared to deliver a shock with minimal delay at the end of the 2-minute cycle of CPR.

Maintain high-quality, uninterrupted chest compressions

The quality of chest compressions and ventilations are important determinants of outcome. Avoid interruptions in chest compressions. Ensure compressions are of adequate depth (5–6 cm) and rate (100–120 min^{-1}), and there is full recoil of the chest at the end of each compression. As soon as the airway is secured, continue chest compressions without pausing during ventilation. To reduce fatigue, change the individual undertaking compressions every 2 minutes or earlier if necessary.

Airway and ventilation

Use a bag-valve-mask with high-flow oxygen, or preferably, a supraglottic airway (SGA) (e.g. i-gel). Once a supraglottic airway has been inserted, attempt to deliver continuous chest compressions, uninterrupted during ventilation. Ventilate the lungs at 10 breaths min^{-1}; do not hyperventilate the lungs.

If excessive gas leakage causes inadequate ventilation of the patient's lungs, chest compressions will need to be interrupted to enable ventilation (using a compression to ventilation ratio of 30:2).

Tracheal intubation should only be attempted by a healthcare provider who is properly trained and has regular, ongoing experience with the technique. Avoid stopping chest compressions during laryngoscopy and intubation; if necessary, a brief pause in chest compressions may be required as the tube is passed between the vocal cords, but this pause should not exceed 5 seconds. Alternatively, to avoid any interruptions in chest compressions, the intubation attempt may be deferred until after ROSC, and will require appropriate intubation medications. After intubation, confirm the correct tube position using waveform capnography and secure it adequately. If the patient's trachea has been intubated, continue chest compressions at a rate of 100–120 min^{-1} without pausing during ventilation.

Monitoring during CPR

Several methods can be used to monitor the patient during CPR and potentially help guide ALS interventions. These include:

- **Clinical signs,** such as breathing efforts, movements and eye opening, can occur during CPR. These can indicate ROSC and require verification by a rhythm and pulse check, but can also occur because high-quality CPR can generate sufficient circulation to restore signs of life, including consciousness.
- **Pulse checks** can be used to identify ROSC when there is an ECG rhythm compatible with a pulse. However, you may not detect pulses in those with low cardiac output states and a low blood pressure. If there is any doubt, start CPR.
- **Monitoring the heart rhythm** through pads is a standard part of ALS. Motion artefacts prevent reliable heart rhythm assessment during chest compressions.
- **End-tidal CO_2** ($ETCO_2$) measured with waveform capnography during CPR is addressed in more detail below.
- **Blood sampling and analysis** during CPR can be used to identify potentially reversible causes of cardiac arrest. Avoid finger prick samples because they may not be reliable; instead, use samples from veins or arteries.
- **Invasive cardiovascular monitoring** in critical care settings (e.g. continuous arterial blood pressure and central venous pressure monitoring). Invasive arterial pressure monitoring will enable the detection of even very low blood pressure values when ROSC is achieved.
- **The use of focused echocardiography/ultrasound** to identify and treat reversible causes of cardiac arrest and identify low cardiac output states ('pseudo-PEA') is discussed below.

Figure 7.6 Intraosseous needle placement into the proximal tibia

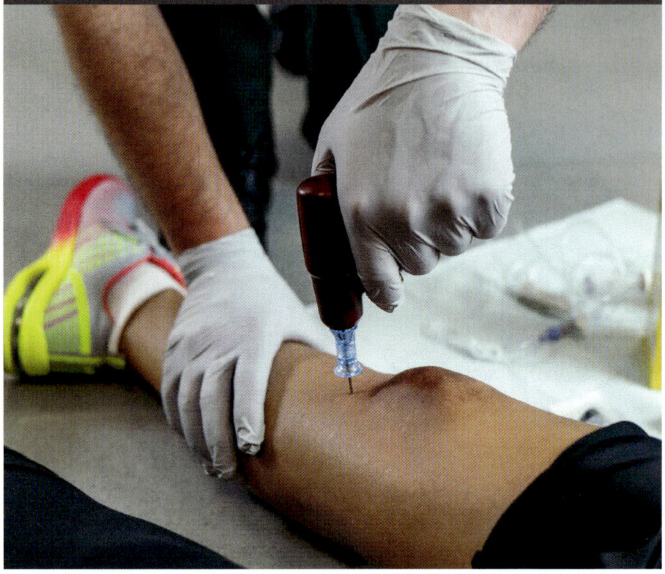

Waveform capnography during advanced life support

Carbon dioxide (CO_2) is a waste product of metabolism; approximately 400 L are produced each day. It is carried in the blood to the lungs, where it is exhaled. End-tidal CO_2 ($ETCO_2$) is the partial pressure of CO_2 at the end of an exhaled breath. It reflects cardiac output and lung blood flow (CO_2 is transported by the venous system to the right side of the heart and then pumped to the lungs by the right ventricle). During CPR, $ETCO_2$ values are low, reflecting the low cardiac output generated by chest compression. Waveform capnography enables continuous, real-time monitoring of $ETCO_2$ during CPR. It works most reliably in patients who have a tracheal tube but can also be used with a supraglottic airway or bag-mask.

The role of waveform capnography during CPR

- Ensuring tracheal tube placement in the trachea. Correct tube placement also relies on observation and auscultation to ensure both lungs are ventilated.
- Monitoring ventilation rate during CPR and avoiding hyperventilation. Monitor the quality of chest compression during CPR. Use $ETCO_2$ values to help monitor the quality of chest compressions and ventilation rates.
- Identifying ROSC during CPR. An increase in $ETCO_2$ during CPR may indicate ROSC and prevent unnecessary and potentially harmful administration of adrenaline in a patient with ROSC. If ROSC is suspected during CPR, withhold adrenaline.
- Prognostication during CPR. Precise values of $ETCO_2$ depend on several factors, including the cause of cardiac arrest, bystander CPR, chest compression quality, ventilation rate and volume, time from cardiac arrest and the use of adrenaline. Low $ETCO_2$ values during CPR are associated with lower rates of ROSC and increased mortality, while high values are associated with better ROSC and survival rates. $ETCO_2$ values should be considered only as part of a multi-modal approach to decision-making for prognostication during CPR.

Vascular access

Some patients will already have intravenous access before they have a cardiac arrest. If this is not the case, ensure CPR has started, and defibrillation, if appropriate, has been attempted before considering vascular access.

Insertion of a central venous catheter requires interruption of CPR and is associated with several potential complications. Peripheral venous cannulation is quicker, easier, and safer. Drugs injected peripherally must be followed by a flush of at least 20 mL of fluid and elevation of the extremity for 10–20 seconds to facilitate drug delivery to the central circulation.

If rapid intravenous access cannot be established after two attempts, consider gaining intraosseous (IO) access (Figure 7.6). The three main insertion sites for IO access during CPR in adults are the proximal humerus, proximal tibia, and distal tibia. Several IO insertion devices are available, ILS providers should be familiar with the one available in their clinical practice setting. Once IO access has been confirmed, resuscitation drugs can be infused.

Fluids and blood products can also be delivered by the IO route, but pressure may be needed to achieve reasonable flow rates using either a pressure bag or a syringe.

Identification and treatment of reversible causes

Potential causes or aggravating factors for which specific treatment exists must be considered during any cardiac arrest. For ease of memory, these are divided into two groups of four based upon their initial letter – either H or T (Figure 7.7):

- **Hypoxia**
- **Hypovolaemia**
- **Hyperkalaemia, hypokalaemia, hypoglycaemia, hypocalcaemia, acidaemia and other metabolic disorders**
- **Hypothermia**
- **Thrombosis (coronary or pulmonary)**
- **Tension pneumothorax**
- **Tamponade – cardiac**
- **Toxins.**

Figure 7.7 The four Hs and four Ts

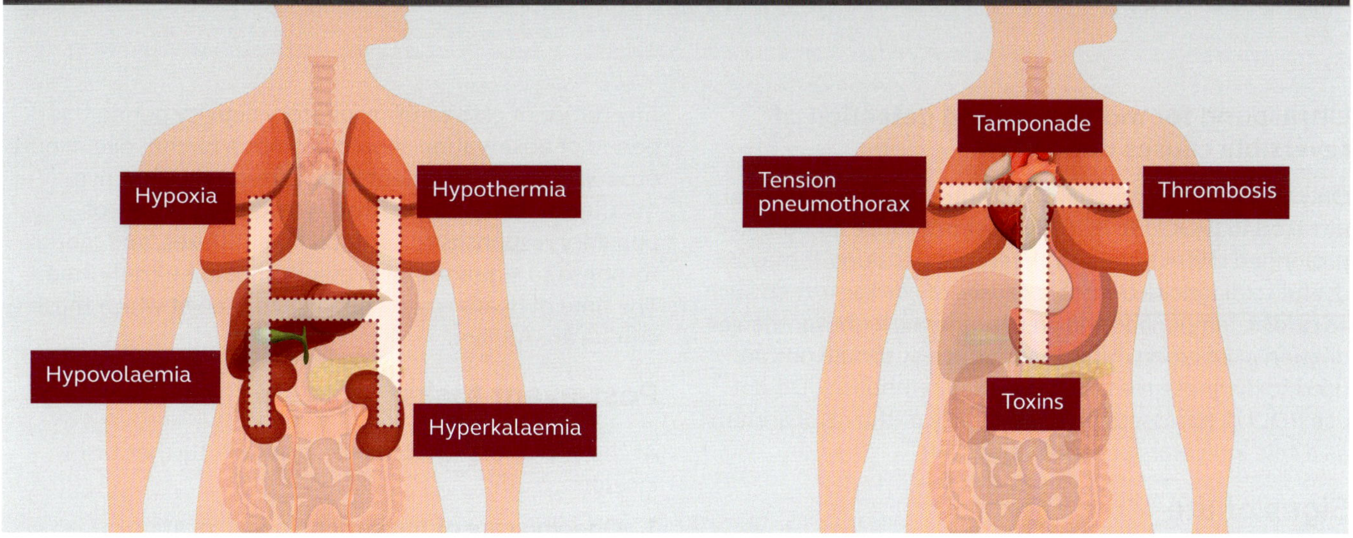

The four Hs

Minimise the risk of **hypoxia** by ensuring that the patient's lungs are ventilated adequately with 100% oxygen during CPR. Check carefully that the SGA is well sited and effective. Ensure the tracheal tube (if used) is not misplaced in a bronchus or the oesophagus.

Pulseless electrical activity caused by **hypovolaemia** is usually due to sepsis or severe bleeding, which can be caused by trauma, gastrointestinal bleeding, or rupture of an aortic aneurysm. Restore intravascular volume rapidly with fluid and, if concerns of bleeding, blood. Obviously, such patients need urgent control of bleeding by surgery or other means (e.g. compression, interventional radiology, tourniquet). Other courses of hypovolaemia can also be present. Effective chest compressions require an adequate circulating volume.

Hyperkalaemia, hypokalaemia, hypoglycaemia, hypocalcaemia, acidaemia and other metabolic disorders are detected by biochemical tests or suggested by the patient's medical history (e.g. renal failure). A 12-lead ECG (performed prior to the cardiac arrest) may help with the diagnosis. Intravenous calcium chloride is indicated in the presence of hyperkalaemia, hypocalcaemia, and calcium channel-blocker overdose.

Hypoglycaemia as a sole reversible cause of cardiac arrest is controversial. A very low blood glucose level, however, can cause irreversible brain damage and should be corrected during CPR. Always measure the blood glucose to exclude hypoglycaemia.

Consider **hypothermia** if appropriate; use a low-reading thermometer.

The four Ts

Coronary **thrombosis** is a common cause of cardiac arrest. If initial resuscitation with advanced life support measures are not successful, in some specialist hospitals, it is feasible to perform percutaneous coronary angiography and percutaneous coronary intervention during ongoing CPR. This usually requires an automated mechanical chest compression device or a heart-bypass type machine (extracorporeal life support) to maintain circulation during the procedure.

The most common cause of thromboembolic or mechanical circulatory obstruction is massive pulmonary embolism. If pulmonary embolism is thought to be the cause of cardiac arrest, consider giving a thrombolytic drug immediately. Out-of-hospital providers should consider early transportation to such specialist units where available, with mechanical CPR.

A tension pneumothorax can cause PEA. The diagnosis is made clinically or by focused ultrasound of the chest. Signs of tension pneumothorax include decreased air entry, decreased expansion, and hyper-resonance to percussion on the affected side, as well as tracheal deviation away from the affected side. Decompress rapidly by thoracostomy or needle thoracocentesis and then insert a chest drain.

Cardiac tamponade is difficult to diagnose because the typical signs of distended neck veins and hypotension cannot be assessed during cardiac arrest. Cardiac arrest after penetrating chest trauma or after cardiac surgery should raise strong suspicion of tamponade – the need for needle pericardiocentesis or resuscitative thoracotomy should be considered.

If there is no specific history of accidental or deliberate ingestion, poisoning by therapeutic or **toxins** (toxic substances) is difficult to detect and may only be shown by laboratory investigations. Where available, the appropriate antidotes should be used; however, treatment is most often supportive.

Ultrasound for monitoring and detection of reversible causes during CPR

Only skilled operators should use intra-arrest point-of-care ultrasound (POCUS). POCUS must not cause additional or prolonged interruptions in chest compressions; it may be useful to diagnose treatable causes of cardiac arrest, such as cardiac tamponade and pneumothorax. Right ventricular dilation in isolation during cardiac arrest should not be used to diagnose massive pulmonary embolism. Do not use POCUS for assessing contractility of the myocardium as a sole indicator for terminating CPR.

Signs of life

If signs of life (such as regular respiratory effort or movement) or readings from patient monitors compatible with ROSC (e.g. a sudden increase in $ETCO_2$ or an arterial blood pressure waveform) appear during CPR, stop CPR briefly and check the monitor. If an organised rhythm is present, check for a pulse. If a pulse is palpable, continue post-resuscitation care. If no pulse is present, continue CPR.

The duration of a resuscitation attempt

If attempts at achieving ROSC are unsuccessful, the resuscitation team leader should discuss stopping CPR with the team. The decision to stop CPR requires clinical judgement and a careful assessment of the likelihood of achieving ROSC and long-term survival. If it is considered appropriate to start resuscitation, it is usually worthwhile to continue, as long as the patient remains in VF/pVT or there is a potentially reversible cause that can be treated.

Diagnosing death after unsuccessful resuscitation

If CPR does not achieve ROSC and a decision is made to discontinue CPR efforts, after stopping CPR, observe the patient for a minimum of five minutes before confirming death. The absence of mechanical cardiac function is normally confirmed using a combination of the following:

- absence of a central pulse on palpation
- absence of heart sounds on auscultation.

One or more of the following can supplement these criteria:

- asystole on a continuous ECG display
- absence of pulsatile flow using direct intra-arterial pressure monitoring
- absence of contractile activity using echocardiography.

Any return of cardiac or respiratory activity during this period of observation should prompt a further five minute observation. If the patient should re-arrest after five minutes of continued cardiac arrest, the absence of pupillary responses to light, corneal reflexes, and motor response to supraorbital pressure should be confirmed. The time of death is recorded as the time at which these criteria are fulfilled.

Post-event tasks

At the end of the resuscitation attempt, further tasks include:

1. **Ongoing care of the patient,** and allocation of further team roles and responsibilities, including handover to other teams.
2. **Documentation of the resuscitation attempt.** Use information from defibrillators and monitors to help document events and times.
3. **Communication with relatives** (Chapter 6). An operational debrief (OD) is led by the clinical team. This is a learning conversation that primarily focuses on the team's performance, i.e., how can we learn from this event and improve our performance next time? An OD can also support responder wellbeing.
4. **Ensuring equipment and drug trolleys are replenished.**
5. **Ensuring audit forms are completed.**
6. **More information about post-resuscitation procedure can be found in Chapter 6.**

RCUK has developed an online resource with more detailed information on the topic of responder wellbeing, available at www.resus.org.uk/responder-wellbeing. See Chapter 6.

SCAN ME for responder wellbeing support

07 SUMMARY LEARNING

The ALS algorithm provides a framework for the standardised resuscitation of all adult patients in cardiac arrest.

The delivery of high-quality chest compressions with minimal interruptions is a crucial determinant of outcome.

Treatment depends on the underlying rhythm.

Look for reversible causes and, if present, treat early.

Secure the airway early to enable continuous chest compressions.

Use waveform capnography to help assess and guide resuscitation interventions.

TEST YOURSELF QUESTIONS

1. What are the reversible causes of cardiac arrest (four Hs and four Ts)?
2. What are the roles of waveform capnography (CO_2 monitoring) during CPR?

My key take-home messages from this chapter are:

Further reading

Academy of Medical Royal Colleges. A code of practice for the diagnosis and confirmation of death. 2010. http://www.aomrc.org.uk

Chrimes, N., Higgs, A., Hagberg, C.A., Baker, P.A., Cooper, R.M., Greif, R., Kovacs, G., Law, J.A., Marshall, S.D., Myatra, S.N., O'Sullivan, E.P., Rosenblatt, W.H., Ross, C.H., Sakles, J.C., Sorbello, M. and Cook, T.M. (2022), Preventing unrecognised oesophageal intubation: a consensus guideline from the Project for Universal Management of Airways and international airway societies*. Anaesthesia, 77: 1395-1415.

Cook TM, Woodall N, Harper J, Benger J; Fourth National Audit Project. Major complications of airway management in the UK: results of the Fourth National Audit Project of the Royal College of Anaesthetists and the Difficult Airway Society. Part 2: intensive care and emergency departments. Br J Anaesth. 2011;106:632-42.

Couper K, Kimani PK, Abella BS, et al. The System-Wide Effect of Real-Time Audiovisual Feedback and Postevent Debriefing for In-Hospital Cardiac Arrest: The Cardiopulmonary Resuscitation Quality Improvement Initiative. Crit Care Med. 2015 Jul 16.

Drennan IR, Greif R, Bray JE, et al., on behalf of the ILCOR Advanced Life Support Task Force. 2025 International Consensus on Cardiopulmonary Resuscitation and Emergency Cardiovascular Care Science With Treatment Recommendations. Advanced Life Support. ILCOR, 2025. In print.

FEEL – Focused Echocardiography in Emergency Life Support www.resus.org.uk/

Gates S, Quinn T, Deakin CD, Blair L, Couper K, Perkins GD. Mechanical chest compression for out-of-hospital cardiac arrest: Systematic review and meta-analysis. Resuscitation 2015;94:91–7.

Nolan JP, Soar J, Smith GB, et al. Incidence and outcome of in- hospital cardiac arrest in the United Kingdom National Cardiac Arrest Audit. Resuscitation 2014;85:987-92.

Soar J, Böttiger B, Carli P, et al. European Resuscitation Council Guidelines 2025: Advanced Life Support. Resuscitation. 2025.In print.

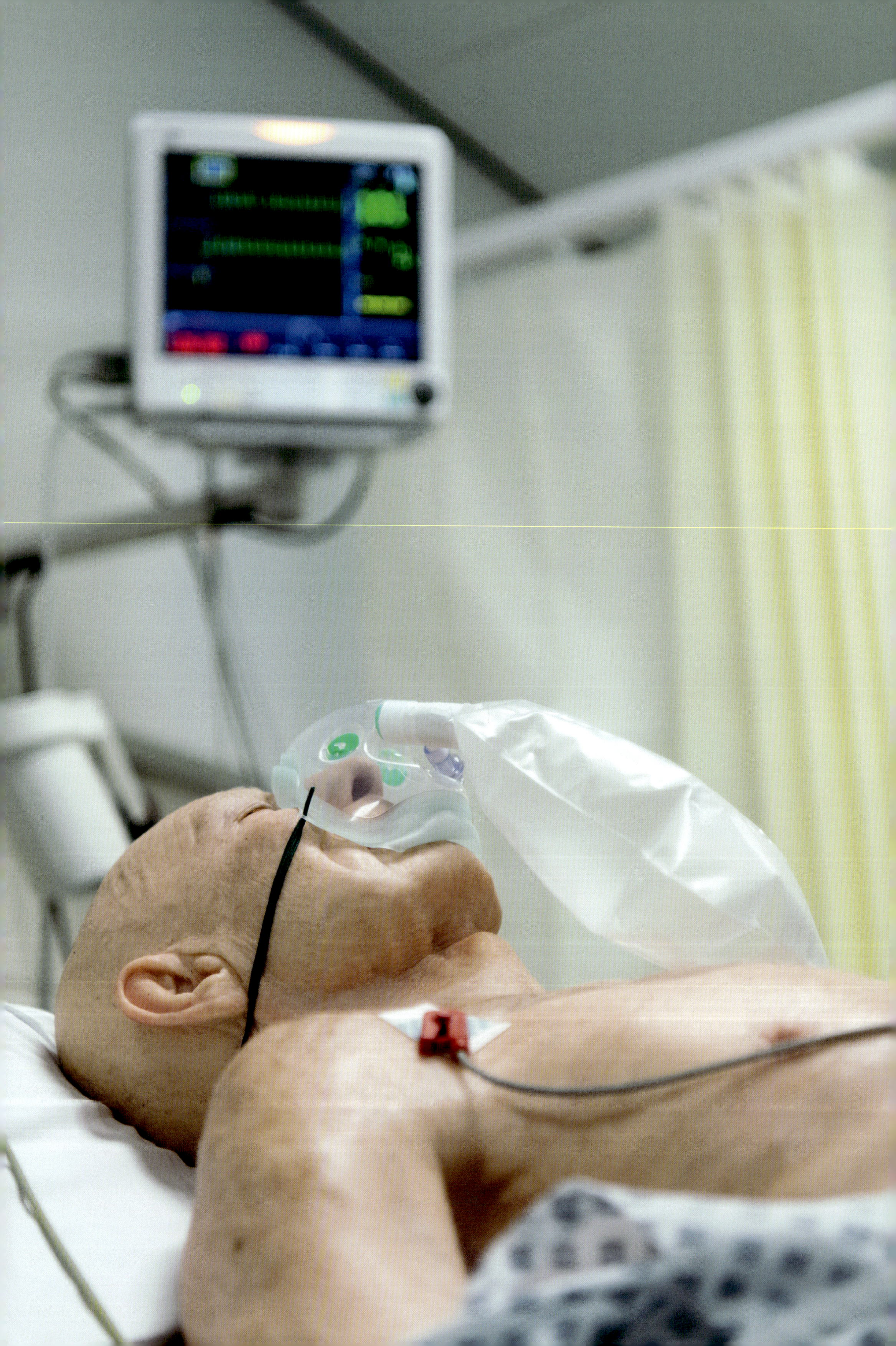

08 Cardiac arrest rhythms – monitoring and recognition

In this chapter

ECG monitoring

Diagnosing cardiac arrest rhythms from cardiac monitors

The learning outcomes will enable you to:

Understand the reasons for ECG monitoring

Monitor the ECG

Recognise the rhythms associated with cardiac arrest

Introduction

ECG monitoring enables identification of the cardiac rhythm in patients in cardiac arrest. Monitoring patients at risk of developing arrhythmias (abnormal heart rhythm) can enable treatment before cardiac arrest occurs.

Patients at risk of cardiac arrest include those with:

- chest pain
- collapse or syncope
- palpitations, or
- shock (e.g. due to bleeding or sepsis).

Basic, single-lead ECG monitoring does not reliably detect cardiac ischemia. Record serial 12-lead ECGs in patients experiencing chest pain suggestive of an acute coronary syndrome. In all patients who have persistent arrhythmia and are at risk of deterioration, cardiac monitoring alone will not always enable accurate rhythm recognition, and it is important to document the arrhythmia in 12-leads for future reference.

Accurate analysis of cardiac rhythm abnormalities requires experience, but by applying basic principles, most rhythms can be interpreted sufficiently to enable selection of the appropriate treatment. The inability to reliably recognise VF/pVT is a major drawback in the use of manual defibrillators.

Automated external defibrillators (AEDs) overcome this problem by automatically analysing the rhythm. For a shockable rhythm, the defibrillator charges to a pre-determined energy and instructs the operator that a shock is required. The introduction of AEDs has meant that more people can now defibrillate safely. People who lack training or confidence in recognising cardiac rhythms should use AEDs.

Accurate analysis of some rhythm abnormalities requires experience and expertise; however, the non-expert can interpret most rhythms sufficiently to identify what immediate treatment is needed. The main priority is to recognise that the rhythm is abnormal and that the heart rate is inappropriately slow or fast. Use the structured approach to rhythm interpretation described in this chapter to help you avoid errors. Any need for immediate treatment will be determined primarily by the effect of the arrhythmia on the patient, rather than by the nature of the arrhythmia itself. When an arrhythmia is present, first assess the patient (use the ABCDE assessment), and then interpret the rhythm as accurately as possible.

Figure 8.1 Electrode positions

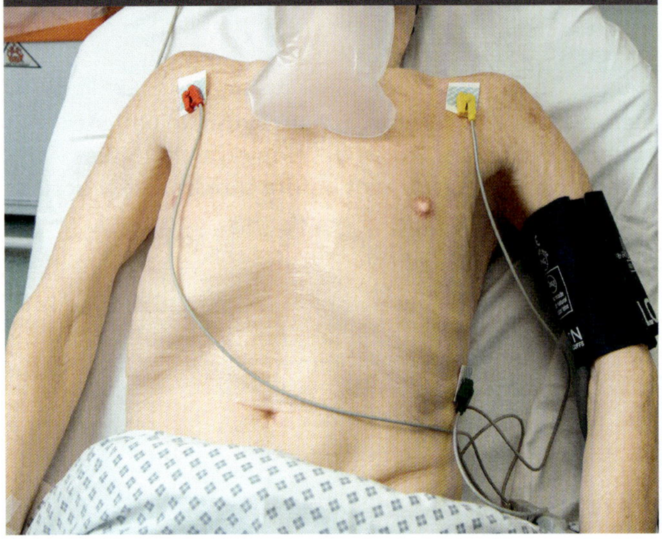

Figure 8.2a Pectoral and apical positions for defibrillator pads

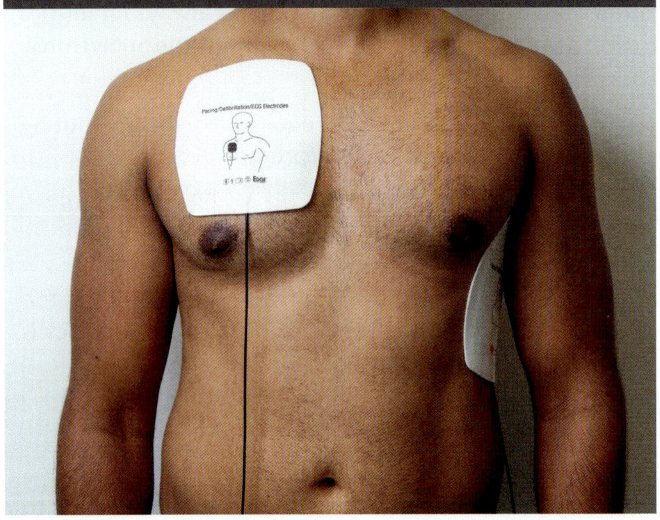

Figure 8.2b Lateral pad placement

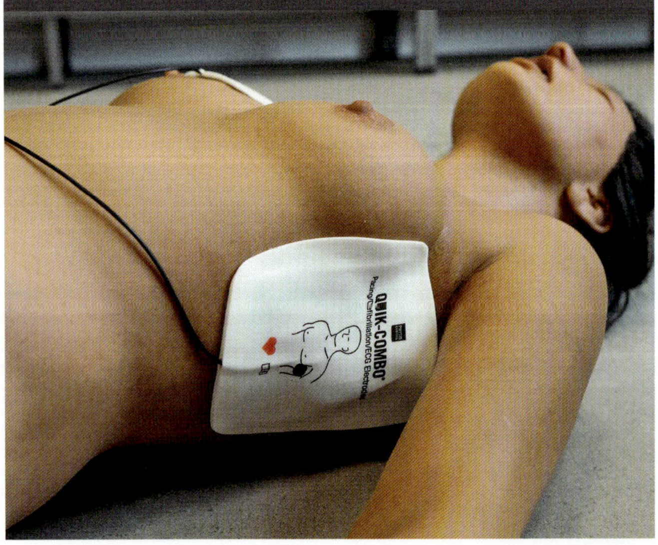

ECG monitoring

Planned ECG monitoring

Attach ECG electrodes to the patient using the positions shown in Figure 8.1. These will enable monitoring using 'modified limb leads' I, II and III.

1. Ensure the skin is dry, not greasy (use an alcohol swab and/or an abrasive pad to clean)
2. Either place the electrodes on relatively hair-free skin or shave off dense hair.
3. Place electrodes over bone rather than muscle to minimise interference in the ECG signal from muscle artefact.

Different electrode positions may be used when necessary (e.g. trauma, recent surgery, skin disease).

Most ECG leads are colour-coded to help with correct connection

The usual colours are:

Red for the Right arm lead
usually placed over the right shoulder joint

yeLLow for the Left arm lead
usually placed over the left shoulder joint

Green for the leG lead
usually placed on the abdomen or lower left chest wall (Figure 8.1).

Begin by monitoring in modified lead II, as this typically displays good amplitude sinus P waves and good amplitude QRS complexes. However, switch to another lead if necessary to obtain the best ECG signal. Try to minimise muscle and movement artefact by explaining to patients what the monitoring is for and by keeping them warm and relaxed.

Emergency monitoring

In an emergency, such as a collapsed patient, assess the cardiac rhythm as soon as possible by applying self-adhesive defibrillator pads in the usual position, as mentioned in Chapter 3 (Figures 8.2a, b, and 8.3). Monitor the cardiac rhythm continuously with proper ECG electrodes as soon as possible after cardiac arrest.

Figure 8.3a, b & c Anterior-posterior (AP) pad positions

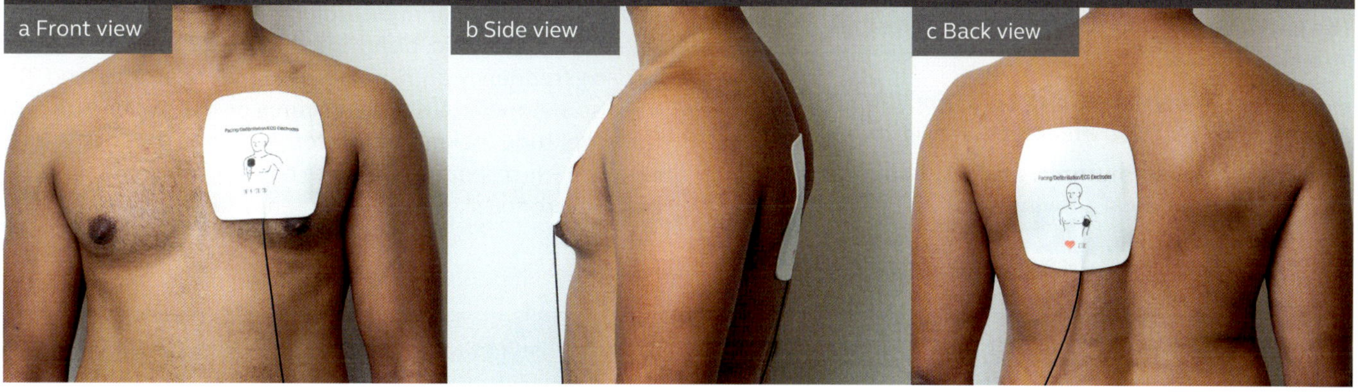

Diagnosis from cardiac monitors

The displays and printouts from cardiac monitors are suitable only for recognising rhythms and not for more detailed ECG interpretation.

Basic electrocardiography

The normal adult heart rate is defined as 60–100 min^{-1}. A rate below 60 min^{-1} is a bradycardia, and a rate of 100 min^{-1} or more is a tachycardia. Under normal circumstances, depolarisation is initiated from a group of specialised pacemaker cells, the sinoatrial (SA) node, in the right atrium (Figure 8.4). The wave of depolarisation spreads from the SA node into the atrial muscle; this is seen on the ECG as the P wave (Figure 8.5). Atrial contraction is the mechanical response to this electrical impulse.

Figure 8.4 Electrical conduction in the heart / cardiac conducting system

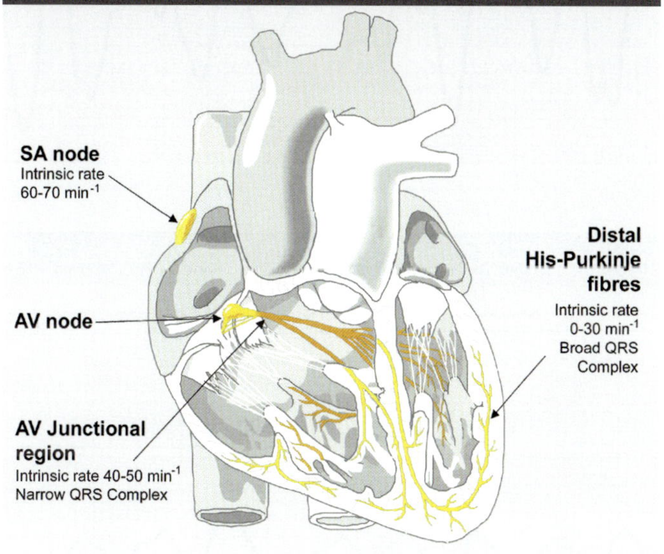

The electrical impulse is spread to the ventricular muscle along specialised conducting tissue through the atrioventricular (AV) node and His-Purkinje system. The bundle of His bifurcates to enable depolarisation to spread into the ventricular muscle along two specialised bundles of conducting tissue, the right bundle branch to the right ventricle, and the left bundle to the left ventricle.

Depolarisation of the ventricles is reflected in the QRS complex of the ECG. The normal sequence of cardiac depolarisation described above is known as sinus rhythm (Rhythm strip 1). The T wave that follows the QRS complex represents ventricular repolarisation. The specialised cells of the conducting tissue (the AV node and His-Purkinje system) enable coordinated ventricular depolarisation, which is more rapid than uncoordinated depolarisation. With normal depolarisation, the QRS complex is narrow, which is defined as less than 0.12 seconds. If one of the bundle branches is diseased, conduction delay causes a broad QRS complex (i.e. greater than 0.12 seconds (3 small squares on the ECG)).

Figure 8.5 Components of the normal ECG signal

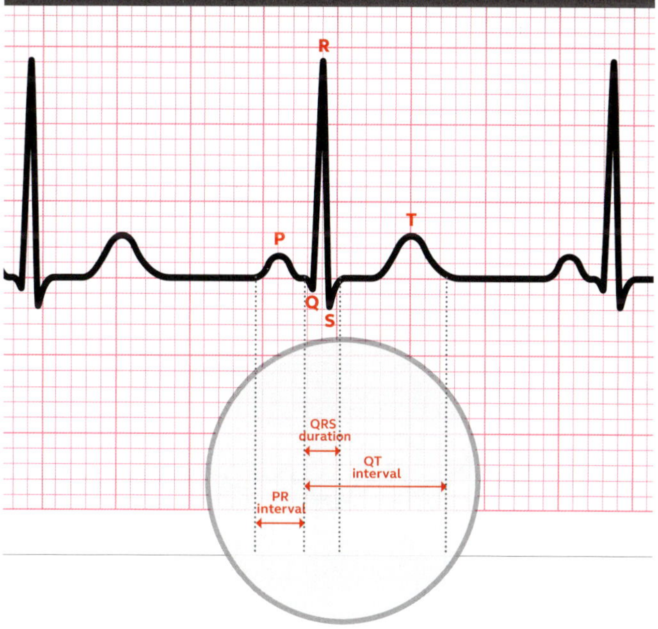

Cardiac arrest rhythms

The rhythms present during cardiac arrest are classified into two groups:

- **Shockable rhythms:** ventricular fibrillation (VF) and pulseless ventricular tachycardia (pVT).
- **Non-shockable rhythms:** asystole and pulseless electrical activity (PEA).

Ventricular fibrillation (VF)

In VF, the ventricular myocardium depolarises randomly. The ECG shows rapid, bizarre, and irregular waves of widely varying frequency and amplitude (Rhythm strips 2 and 3). VF is sometimes classified as coarse or fine depending on the amplitude (height) of the complexes. If the rhythm is clearly VF (irrespective if coarse or fine), attempt defibrillation.

Rhythm strip 1 Example of sinus rhythm

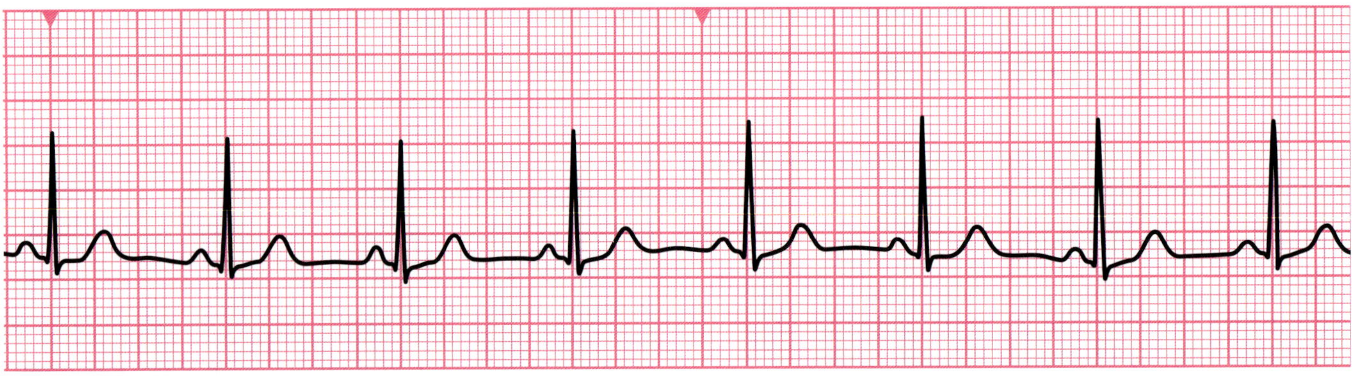

Rhythm strip 2 Ventricular fibrillation (VF) shows rapid, bizarre, and irregular waves of widely varying frequency and amplitude

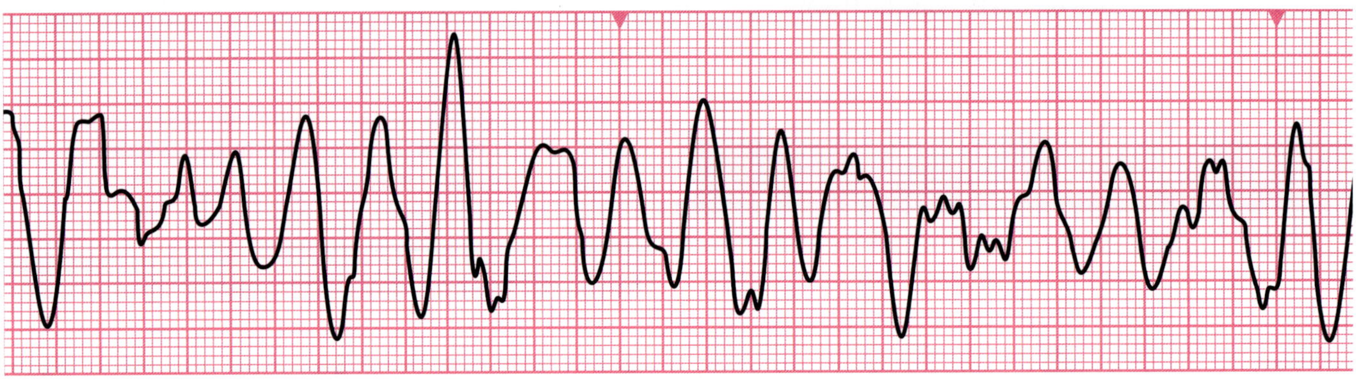

Rhythm strip 3 Fine ventricular fibrillation

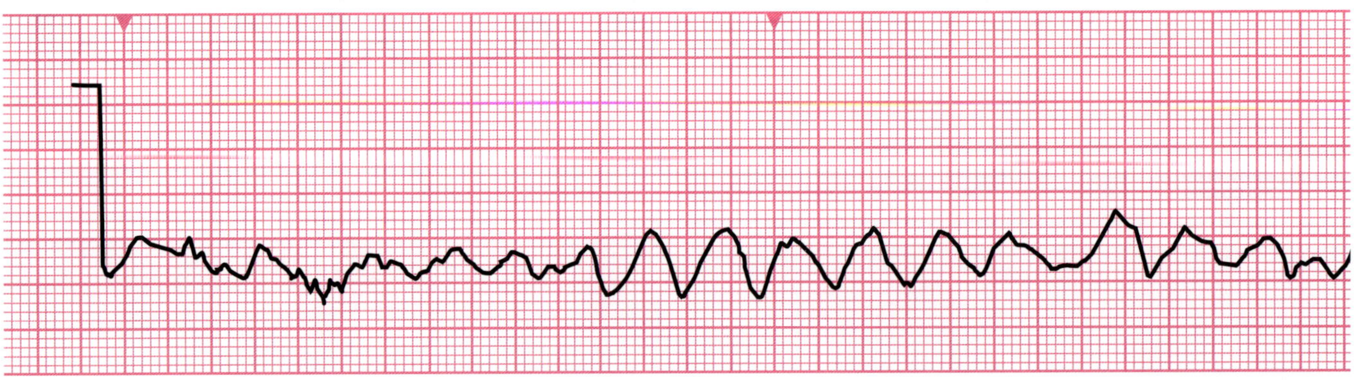

Pulseless ventricular tachycardia (pVT)

Ventricular tachycardia, particularly at higher rates or when the left ventricle is compromised, may cause profound loss of cardiac output. Pulseless VT is managed in the same way as VF. The ECG shows a broad-complex tachycardia. In monomorphic VT, the rhythm is regular (or almost regular) at a rate of 100–300 min^{-1} (Rhythm strip 4).

Asystole

Usually, there is neither atrial nor ventricular activity, and the ECG is more of a straight line (Rhythm strip 5).

Deflections that can be confused with very fine VF can be caused by baseline drift, electrical interference, respiratory movements, or cardiopulmonary resuscitation. A completely straight line usually means that a monitoring lead has disconnected. Whenever asystole is suspected, check that the monitor gain is set correctly and that the leads are connected properly. If the monitor has the facility, view another lead configuration.

Rhythm strip 4 Ventricular tachycardia (VT) shows the rhythm is regular (or almost regular) at a rate of 100–300 min^{-1}

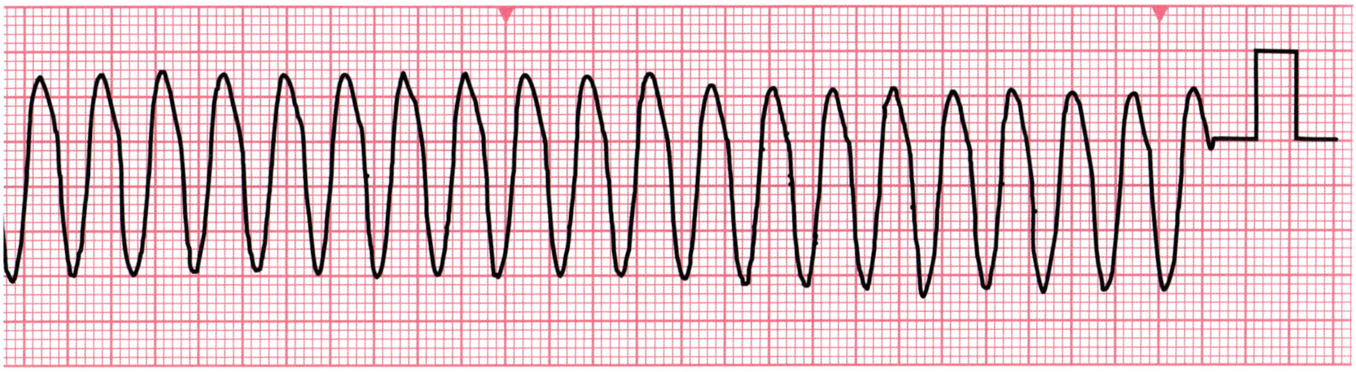

Rhythm strip 5 Asystole – neither atrial nor ventricular activity is present

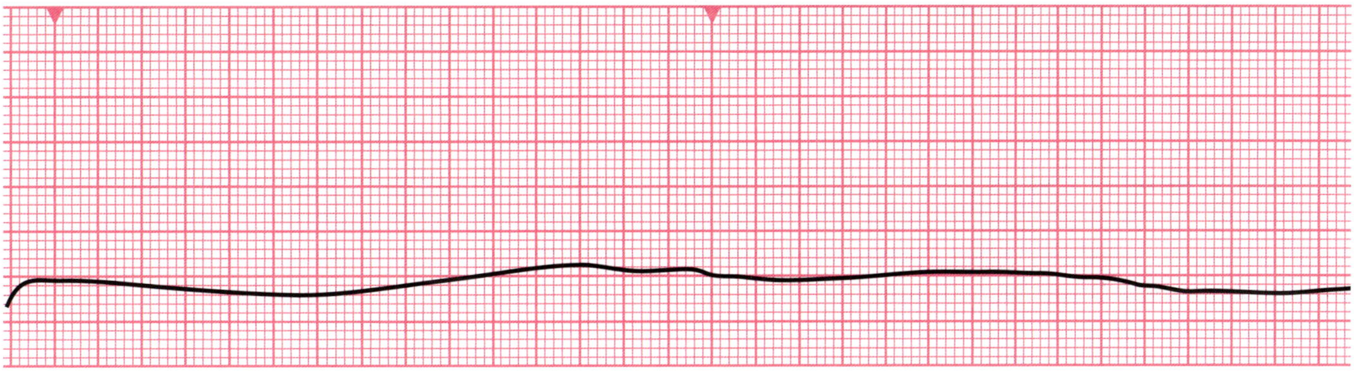

Atrial activity (i.e. P waves) may continue for a short time after the onset of ventricular asystole (ventricular standstill); there will be P waves on the ECG but no evidence of ventricular depolarisation (Rhythm strip 6). These patients may be suitable for cardiac pacing. This is typically referred to as P wave asystole.

Pulseless electrical activity (PEA)

The term pulseless electrical activity (PEA) does not refer to a specific cardiac rhythm. It defines the clinical absence of cardiac output despite the presence of electrical activity that would normally be expected to produce a cardiac output.

Potentially treatable causes include severe fluid depletion or blood loss, cardiac tamponade, massive pulmonary embolism and tension pneumothorax.

Rhythm strip 6 P wave asystole (ventricular standstill with continuing sinus P waves)

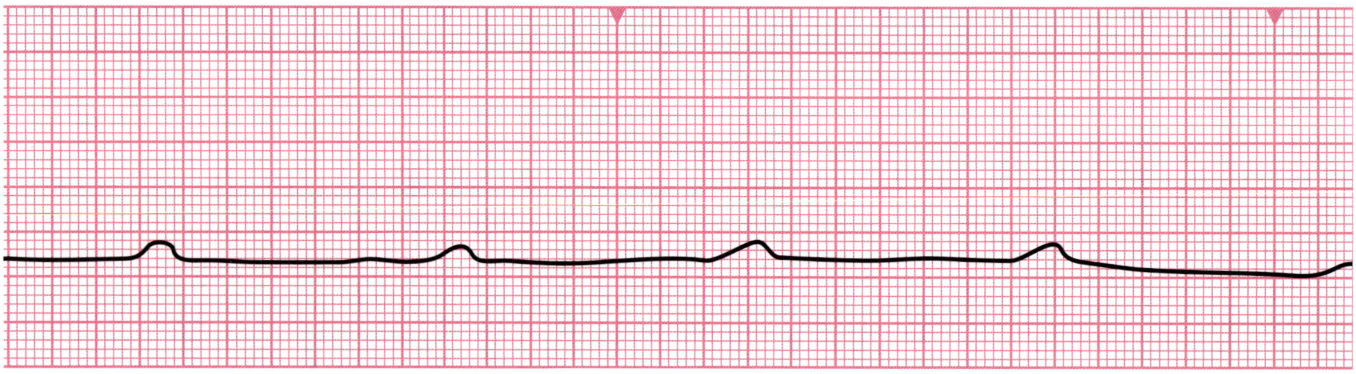

Rhythm strip 7 Sinus bradycardia shows as a slow heart rate of less than 60 min^{-1}

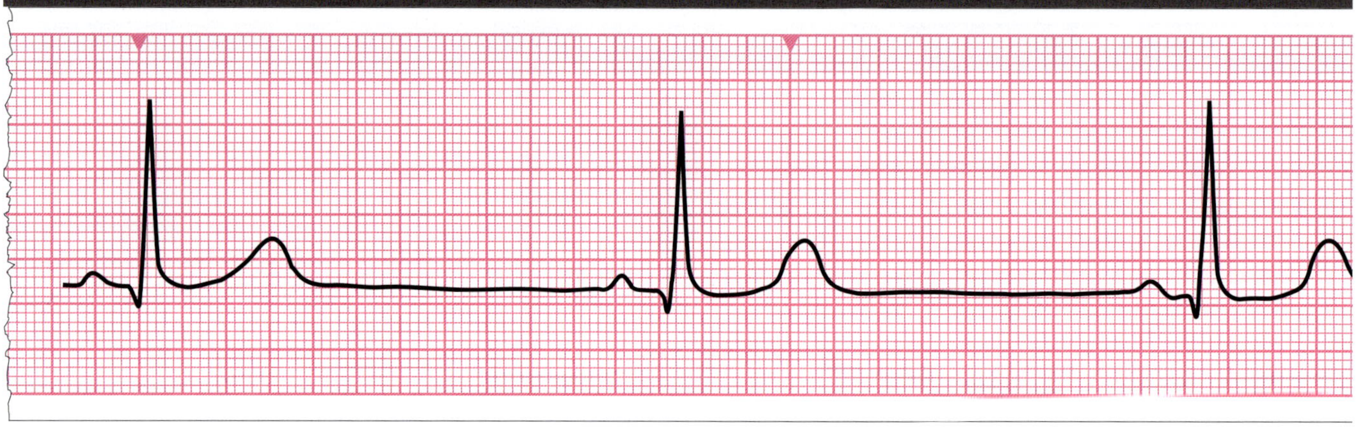

Rhythm strip 8 Agonal rhythm shows as a slow, irregular, wide ventricular complexes of varying shape

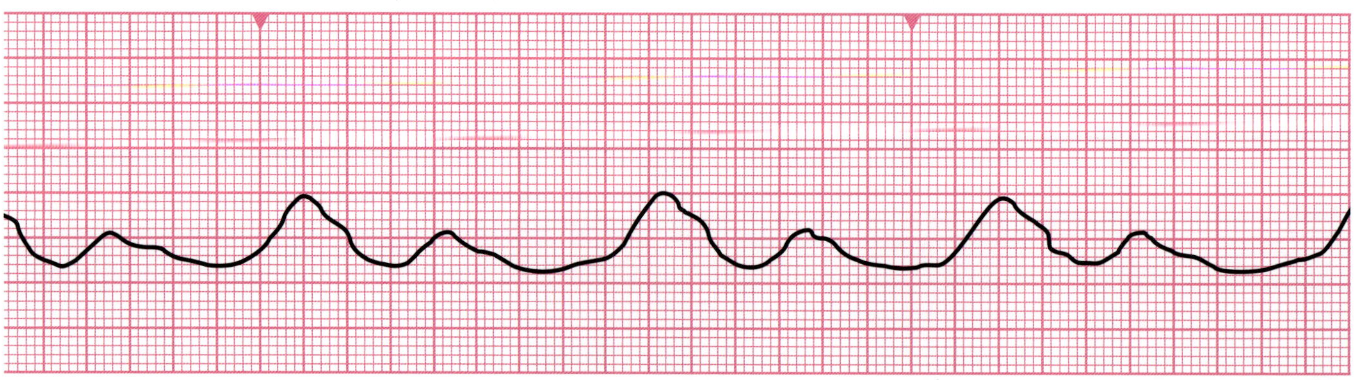

Bradycardia

The treatment of bradycardia (a slow heart rate of less than 60 min^{-1}) (Rhythm strip 7) depends on its haemodynamic consequences. Very slow rates can cause the blood pressure to fall. It is not a true cardiac arrest rhythm, as patients usually have a pulse. Bradycardia may, however, mean imminent cardiac arrest and needs to be treated with atropine or other measures (e.g. pacing) in patients with adverse features (e.g. low blood pressure, fainting (syncope), chest pain, heart failure).

Agonal rhythm

Agonal rhythm occurs in dying patients. Agonal rhythm is characterised by slow, irregular, wide ventricular complexes of varying shape (Rhythm strip 8). This does not generate a pulse. It is usually seen during the late stages of unsuccessful resuscitation. The complexes inevitably slow, becoming progressively broader until all recognisable electrical activity is lost.

08 SUMMARY LEARNING

- Monitor the ECG in all patients in cardiac arrest or at risk of deterioration.
- Automated external defibrillators (AEDs) will recognise shockable rhythms (VF/pVT) and advise a shock.

TEST YOURSELF QUESTIONS

1. Where do you place the electrode leads in 3-lead monitoring?
2. What are the shockable rhythms?
3. What does VF look like on a rhythm strip?

My key take-home messages from this chapter are:

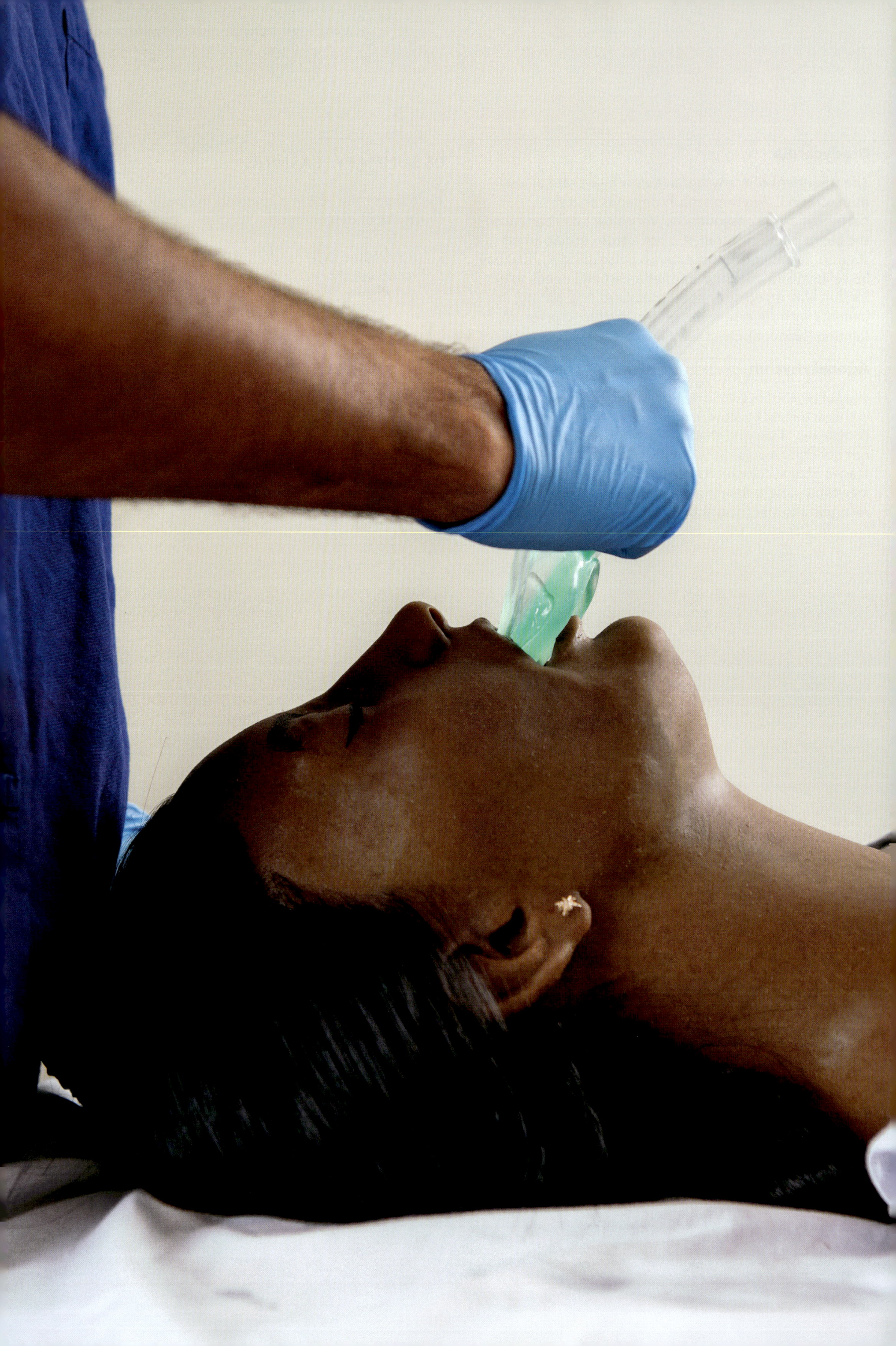

09 Airway management and ventilation

In this chapter

- Causes and recognition of airway obstruction
- Techniques for airway management for the deteriorating patient and resuscitation
- The use of simple adjuncts to maintain airway patency
- Techniques for ventilating the lungs

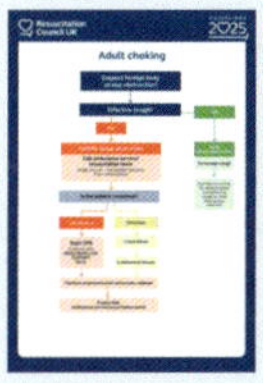

The adult choking algorithm

The learning outcomes will enable you to:

- Recognise the causes of airway obstruction
- Recognise and treat choking
- Use basic airway opening techniques
- Understand the role of the bag-mask ventilation
- Understand the role of supraglottic airways

Introduction

Patients requiring resuscitation often have an obstructed airway, usually caused by loss of consciousness, but occasionally, obstruction is the primary cause of cardiac arrest. Prompt assessment, airway opening, and ventilation are essential to help prevent secondary hypoxic damage to the brain and other vital organs. Without adequate oxygenation, an arrested heart may not restart.

These principles may not apply to witnessed primary cardiac arrest in the vicinity of a defibrillator; in such cases, the priority is immediate defibrillation followed by attention to the airway.

Causes of airway obstruction

Obstruction may be partial or complete. It may occur at any level from the nose and mouth down to the level of the trachea and bronchi.

In the unconscious patient, the most common site of airway obstruction is the pharynx, more often at the soft palate and epiglottis rather than the tongue. Obstruction can also be caused by vomit or blood, by regurgitation of gastric contents, by trauma to the airway, or by foreign bodies. Laryngeal obstruction can be caused by oedema resulting from burns, inflammation, or anaphylaxis.

Upper airway stimulation, or an inhaled foreign body, can cause laryngeal spasm (laryngospasm). Obstruction of the airway below the larynx is less common, but may be caused by excessive bronchial secretions, mucosal oedema, bronchospasm, pulmonary oedema, or aspiration of gastric contents. Extrinsic compression of the airway may also occur above or below the larynx (e.g. trauma, haematoma or tumour).

Recognition of airway obstruction

Recognition is best achieved by the 'look, listen, and feel' approach:

- Look for chest and abdominal movements.
- Listen and feel for airflow at the mouth and nose.

In partial airway obstruction, air entry is diminished and usually noisy:

- Inspiratory stridor or crowing caused by obstruction at the larynx or above, or laryngeal spasm.
- Expiratory wheeze suggests obstruction of the lower airways, which tend to collapse and obstruct during expiration.
- Gurgling suggests there is liquid or semisolid material in the upper airways.
- Snoring arises when the pharynx is partially occluded by the tongue or palate.

During normal breathing, the abdomen is pushed out as the chest wall expands. In contrast, if the airway is obstructed, the abdomen is seen to be pushed out as the chest is drawn in during attempts to inspire. This is often described as 'see-saw breathing'. If the airway is obstructed, the accessory muscles of respiration are used; the neck and shoulder muscles contract to assist in the movement of the thoracic cage. There may also be intercostal and subcostal recession. A full examination of the neck, chest, and abdomen is necessary to differentiate these paradoxical movements from normal breathing.

It is sometimes very difficult, and you must listen for the absence of breath sounds to diagnose complete airway obstruction. When listening, remember that normal breathing should be quiet; obstructed breathing will be silent, but noisy breathing indicates partial airway obstruction. Unless obstruction is relieved to allow adequate ventilation within a very few minutes, neurological and other vital organ injury will occur, leading to cardiac arrest.

Whenever possible, give high-concentration oxygen during the attempt to relieve airway obstruction. Arterial blood oxygen saturation (SaO_2) measurements (normally using pulse oximetry (SpO_2)) will guide further use of oxygen as airway patency improves. If airway patency remains poor and SaO_2 remains low, continue to give high-concentration oxygen. As airway patency improves, blood oxygen saturation values will be restored more rapidly if the inspired oxygen concentration is initially high. Inspired oxygen concentrations can then be adjusted to maintain an SpO_2 at 94–98% or 88–92% for patients with hypercapnic respiratory failure.

Choking

Recognition of choking

Foreign bodies may cause either mild or severe airway obstruction. The signs and symptoms enabling differentiation between mild and severe airway obstruction are summarised in Table 9.1.

Table 9.1 Signs of choking

General signs of choking	
Attack occurs while eating	
Patient may clutch their neck	
Signs of severe airway obstruction	
Response to question 'Are you choking?'	Patient unable to speak
	Patient may respond by nodding
Other signs	Patient unable to breathe
	Breathing sounds wheezy
	Attempts at coughing are silent
	Patient may be unconscious
Signs of mild airway obstruction	
Response to question 'Are you choking?'	Patient speaks and answers yes
Other signs	Patient is able to speak, cough and breathe

Sequence for the treatment of adult choking

1. If the patient shows signs of mild airway obstruction (Figure 9.1)

- Encourage them to continue coughing and monitor the patient's condition.

2. If the patient shows signs of severe airway obstruction and is conscious:

- Give up to 5 back blows.
  - Stand to the side and slightly behind the patient.
  - Support the chest with one hand and lean the patient well forwards.
  - Give up to 5 sharp blows between the scapulae with the heel of the other hand.
- Check to see if each back blow has relieved the airway obstruction.
- If 5 back blows fail to relieve the airway obstruction, give up to 5 abdominal thrusts.
  - Stand behind the patient and put both arms around the upper part of their abdomen.
  - Place a clenched fist just under the xiphisternum; grasp this hand with your other hand and pull sharply inwards and upwards.
  - Repeat up to 5 times.
- If the obstruction is still not relieved, continue alternating 5 back blows with abdominal thrusts.

3. If the patient becomes unconscious

- Call the resuscitation team and start CPR.
- As soon as an individual with appropriate skills is present, look with a laryngoscope and attempt to remove any foreign body with Magill's forceps.

Basic techniques

Opening the airway

Once airway obstruction is recognised, take immediate action to relieve the obstruction and maintain a clear airway. Three manoeuvres can be used to relieve upper airway obstruction:

- **head tilt**
- **chin lift**
- **jaw thrust.**

Adult choking

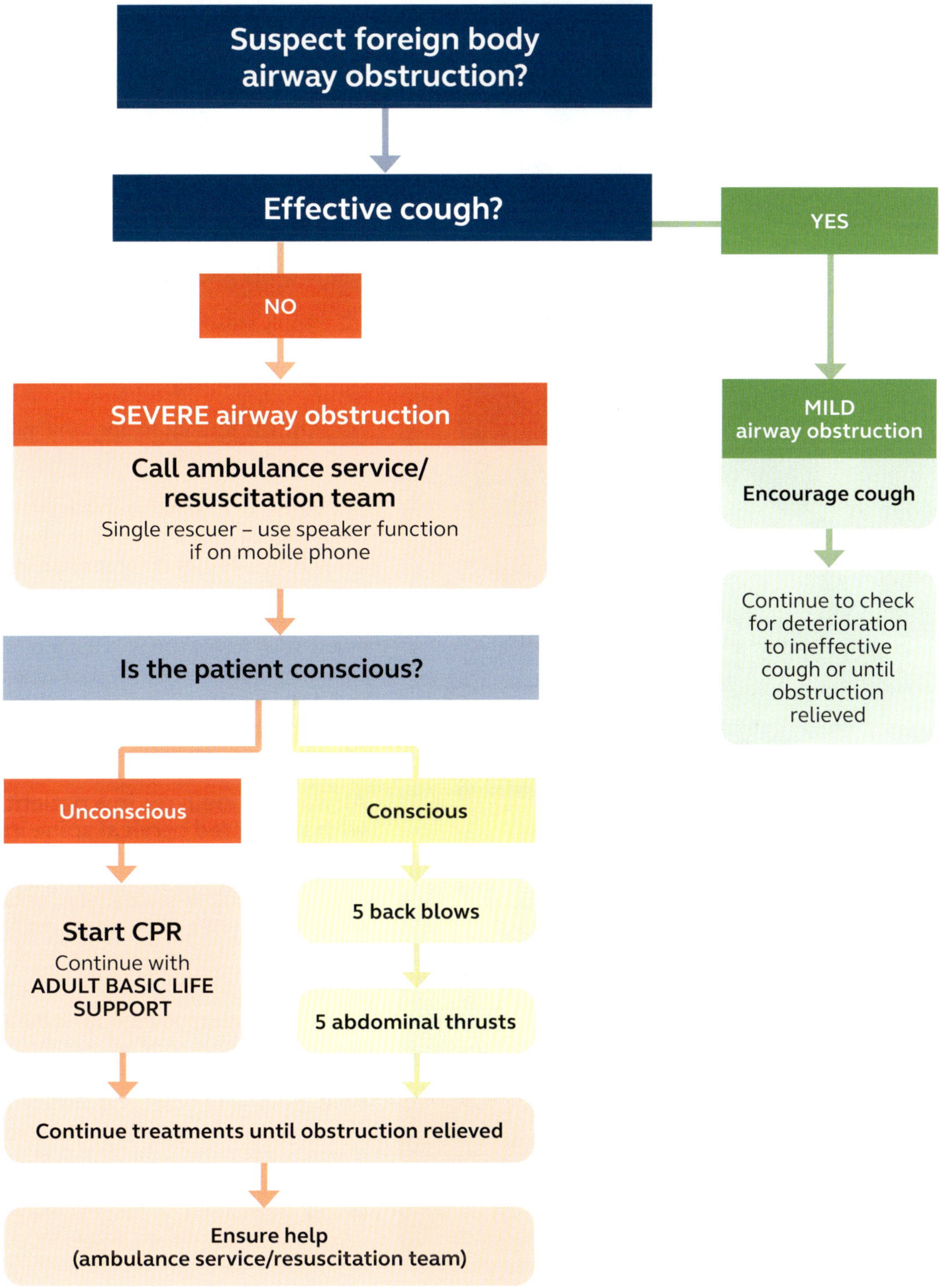

Figure 9.1 Adult choking algorithm

Figure 9.2 Head tilt and chin lift

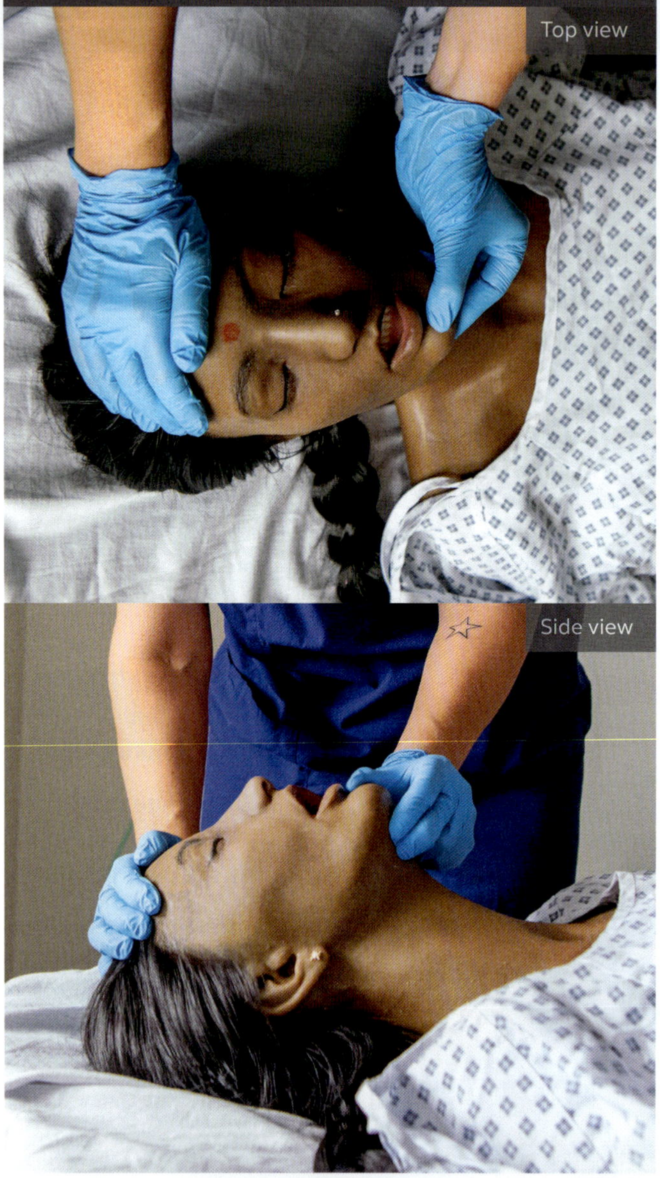

Head tilt and chin lift

Place one hand on the patient's forehead and tilt the head back gently. Place the fingertips of the other hand under the point of the patient's chin and gently lift to stretch the anterior neck structures (Figure 9.2).

Jaw thrust

Jaw thrust is another manoeuvre for bringing the mandible forward and relieving obstruction (Figure 9.3). It is most successful when applied with a head tilt.

Technique for jaw thrust

1. Identify the angle of the mandible.
2. Apply steady upward and forward (anterior) pressure with the index and other fingers placed behind the angle of the mandible.
3. Use the thumbs to open the mouth slightly by downward displacement of the chin.

Jaw thrust, or head tilt and chin lift, will usually clear the airway when the obstruction is caused by relaxation of the soft tissues. Check for success by using the 'look, listen, and feel' sequence described on the previous page. If the airway remains obstructed, inspect and remove any visible solid foreign body in the mouth using forceps or suction. Remove broken or displaced dentures, but leave well-fitting dentures in place, as they help maintain the mouth's contours, which improves the seal for ventilation when using mouth-to-mask or bag-mask techniques.

Airway manoeuvres in a patient with suspected cervical spine injury

If spinal injury is suspected (e.g. if the individual has fallen, been struck on the head or neck, or has been rescued after diving into shallow water), maintain the head, neck, chest, and lumbar region in the neutral position during resuscitation.

Excessive head tilt could worsen the injury and damage the cervical spinal cord; however, this complication remains theoretical, and the relative risk is unknown. When there is a risk of cervical spine injury, establish a clear upper airway by using jaw thrust or chin lift in combination with manual in-line stabilisation of the head and neck by an assistant. If a life-threatening airway obstruction persists despite jaw thrust or chin lift, add a small head tilt at a time until the airway is open; establishing an airway and breathing takes priority over concerns about a potential cervical spine injury.

Figure 9.3 Jaw thrust

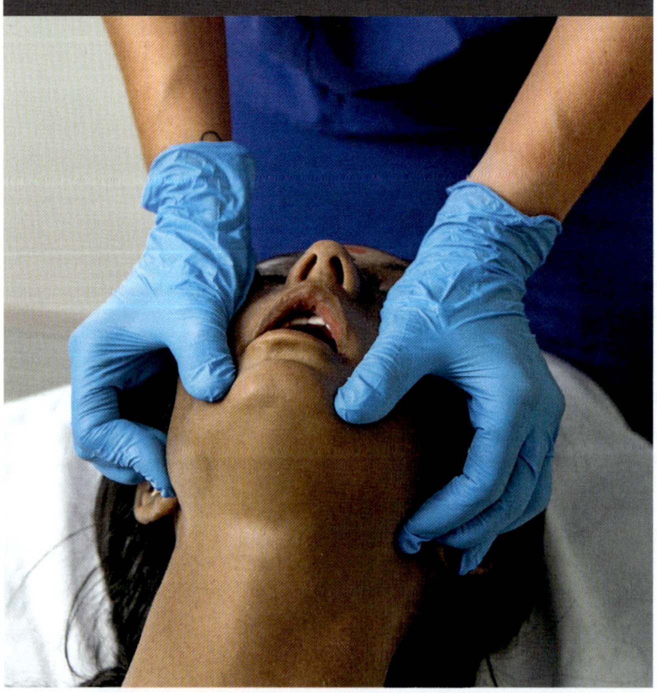

Adjuncts to basic airway techniques

Simple airway adjuncts are often helpful and sometimes essential for maintaining an open airway, particularly when resuscitation is prolonged. Oropharyngeal and nasopharyngeal airways overcome soft palate obstruction and backward tongue displacement in an unconscious patient, but head tilt and jaw thrust may also be necessary.

Oropharyngeal airway

The oropharyngeal (Guedel) airway is a curved plastic tube, flanged and reinforced at the oral end and flattened to fit neatly between the tongue and hard palate (Figure 9.4). There are sizes suitable for small and large adults. Estimate the size by selecting an airway with a length equal to the vertical distance between the patient's incisors and the angle of the jaw (Figure 9.5). The most common sizes are ISO 8.0 (previously labelled as size 2) for small, ISO 9.0 (previously labelled as size 3) for medium, and ISO 10.0 (previously labelled as size 4) for large adults. An airway that is slightly too big will be more beneficial than one that is slightly too small.

Oropharyngeal airways are intended only for unconscious patients; attempted insertion in semi-comatose patients may provoke vomiting or laryngospasm. If a patient is intolerant of an oral airway, they do not need one.

Technique for insertion of an oropharyngeal airway

1. Open the patient's mouth and ensure that there is nothing in the mouth that could be pushed into the larynx; use suction if necessary.
2. Introduce the airway past the teeth or gums 'upside-down' and then rotate it through 180° as it passes beyond the hard palate and into the oropharynx (Figure 9.6). This manoeuvre lessens the chance of pushing the tongue backwards and downwards. Be careful not to lever the front incisors.
3. The patient must be sufficiently obtunded not to gag or strain. If any reflex responses are seen, remove the airway. If the placement is correct, the obstruction will be relieved, and the flattened reinforced section will fit neatly between the patient's front teeth or gums.
4. After insertion, check the airway by the Look, Listen and Feel approach, while maintaining alignment of the head and neck with head tilt, chin lift or jaw thrust as necessary.

Figure 9.4 Oropharyngeal and nasopharyngeal airways

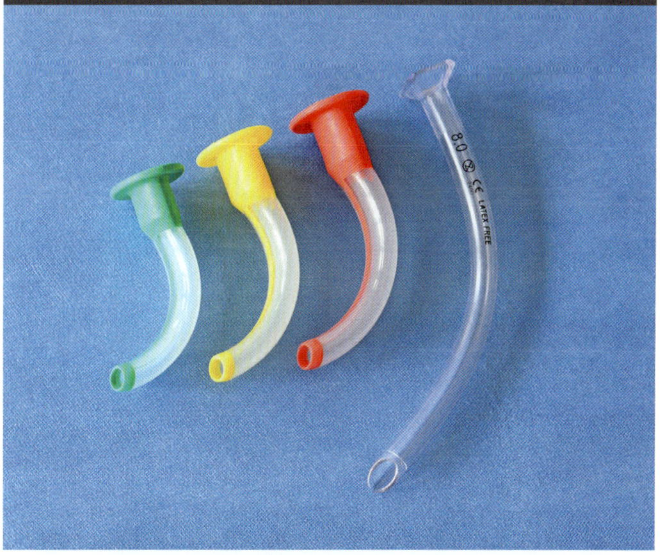

Figure 9.5 Sizing an oropharyngeal airway

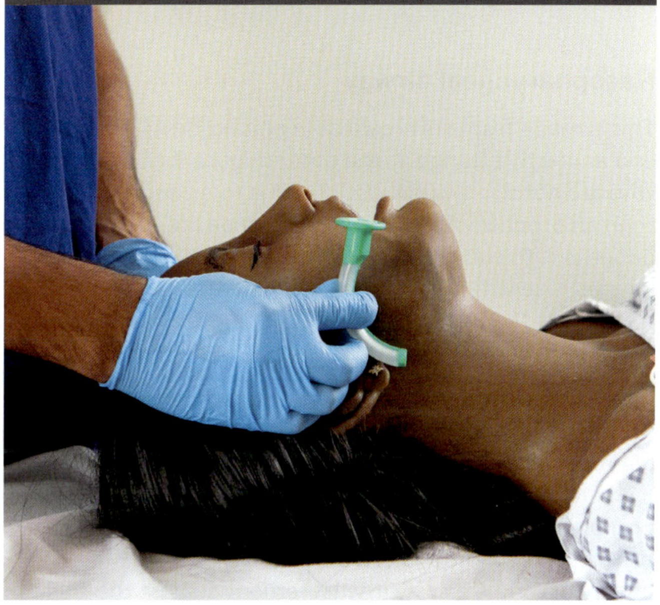

Figure 9.6 Oral airway insertion

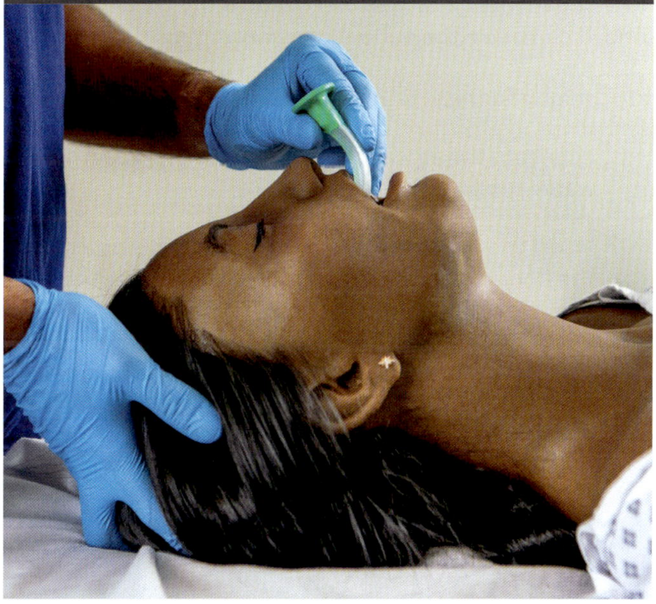

Figure 9.7 Nasopharyngeal airway insertion

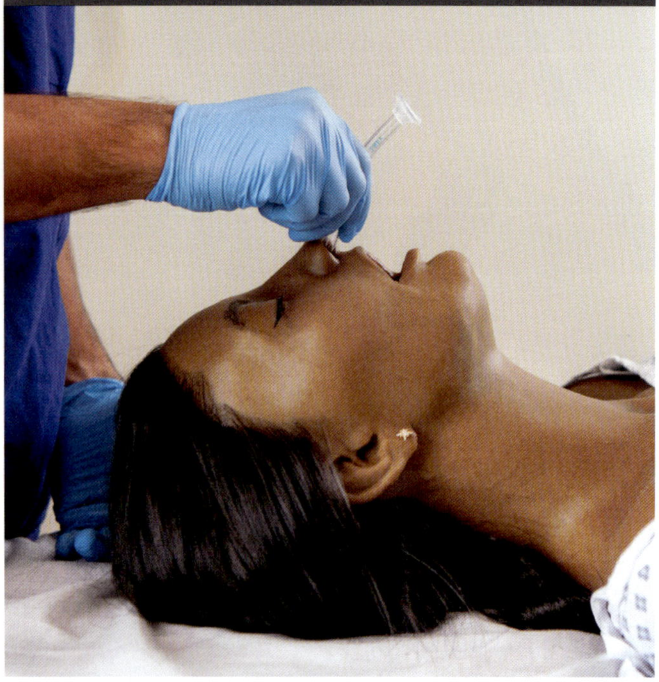

Figure 9.8 Suctioning

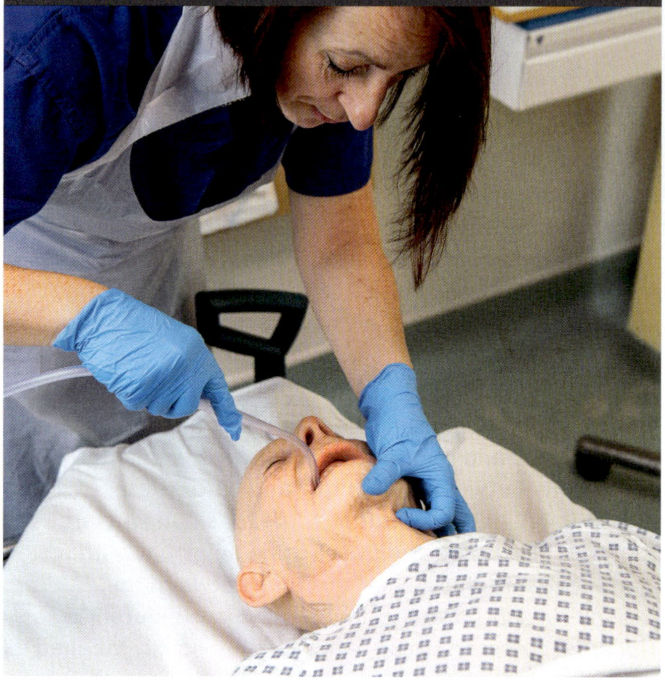

Nasopharyngeal airway

This is made from soft malleable plastic, bevelled at one end and with a flange at the other (Figure 9.4). In patients who are not deeply unconscious, it is tolerated better than an oropharyngeal airway. It may be life-saving in patients with clenched jaws, trismus or maxillofacial injuries. Use with caution in patients with a suspected fracture of the base of skull, and remember they often cause bleeding inside the nose.

The tubes are sized in millimetres according to their internal diameter, and the length increases with diameter. Sizes 6–7 mm are suitable for adults. If the tube is too long, it may stimulate the laryngeal or glossopharyngeal reflexes and cause laryngospasm or vomiting. Traditional methods of sizing a nasopharyngeal airway (measurement against the patient's little finger or anterior nares) are unreliable.

Be careful if you use a nasopharyngeal airway. About 30% of patients get a nosebleed, and if the tube is too long, it can make the patient gag and vomit.

Technique for insertion of a nasopharyngeal airway

1. Lubricate the airway thoroughly using water-soluble jelly.
2. Insert the airway bevel end first, vertically along the floor of the nose with a slight twisting action (Figure 9.7). Try the right nostril first. If any obstruction is met, try the left nostril.
3. Once in place, check for patency and ventilation by look, listen, and feel, and if necessary, maintain correct alignment of the head and neck with chin lift or jaw thrust techniques.

Oxygen

During cardiac arrest, ventilate the lungs with the highest possible oxygen concentration until return of spontaneous circulation (ROSC) is achieved. After ROSC is achieved, administer high-flow oxygen to any acutely ill or unconscious patient until the oxygen saturation of arterial blood (SaO_2) can be reliably measured with pulse oximetry (SpO_2). A low blood oxygen level (hypoxaemia) is harmful, and after ROSC, if hyperventilation occurs, a high blood oxygen level (hyperoxaemia) can also be harmful. A standard oxygen mask (e.g. Hudson mask) will deliver up to 50% inspired oxygen, provided the flow of oxygen is high enough. Initially, give the highest possible oxygen concentration via a mask with a reservoir bag (non-rebreathing mask). This can deliver an inspired oxygen concentration of 85% at flows of 10–15 L min^{-1}. Monitor oxygen saturation using a pulse oximeter (SpO_2) or arterial blood gases to enable titration of the inspired oxygen concentration. When blood oxygen saturation can be measured reliably, oxygen saturations should be maintained between 94–98% or between 88–92% if the patient has hypercapnic respiratory failure.

Suction

Use a wide-bore rigid sucker (Yankauer) to remove liquid (blood, saliva and gastric contents) from the upper airway (Figure 9.8). Be careful if the patient has an intact gag reflex; suction can provoke vomiting. Fine-bore flexible suction catheters can be used in patients with limited mouth opening. They can also be passed through oropharyngeal or nasopharyngeal airways. ILS providers should be familiar with the use of portable suction equipment in their area of practice. Thick vomit can be difficult to suction without a large bore sucker and good suction. Large chunks of food may have to be removed by hand or Magill's forceps.

Figure 9.9 The two-person technique for bag-mask ventilation during CPR

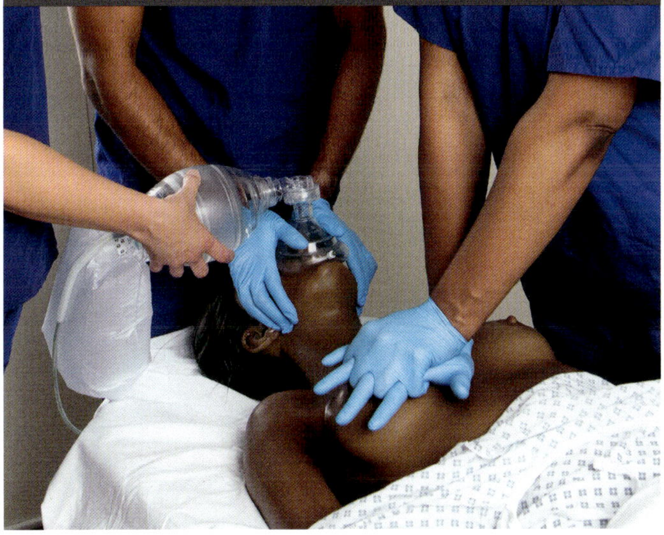

Figure 9.10 i-gel

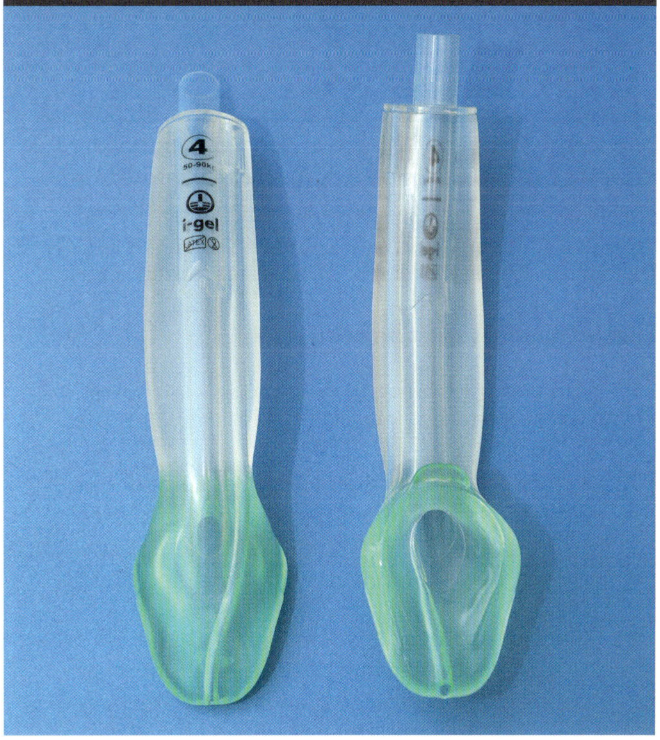

Ventilation

Patients with no, or inadequate, breathing require artificial ventilation. Expired air ventilation (rescue breathing with mouth-to-mouth or mouth-to-mask breaths) is effective, but the rescuer's expired oxygen concentration is only 16–17%, so it must be replaced as soon as possible by ventilation with oxygen-enriched air. Mouth-to-mouth ventilation does not require any equipment but is unpleasant, particularly when vomit or blood is present. There are simple adjuncts for avoiding direct person-to-person contact.

Self-inflating bag

The self-inflating bag can be connected to a face mask (bag-valve mask), a supraglottic airway (e.g. i-gel), or a tracheal tube. As the bag is squeezed, the contents are delivered to the patient's lungs. Upon release, the expired gas is diverted to the atmosphere through a one-way valve; the bag then refills automatically via an inlet at the opposite end.

When used without supplemental oxygen, the self-inflating bag ventilates the patient's lungs with ambient air only (oxygen concentration 21%). This is increased to around 45% by attaching high-flow oxygen directly to the bag adjacent to the air intake. An inspired oxygen concentration of approximately 85% is achieved if a reservoir system is attached and the oxygen flow is high (10–15 L min^{-1}).

A self-inflating bag enables ventilation with high concentrations of oxygen, but its use requires skill and expertise. When used with a face mask, it is difficult to achieve a gas-tight seal while simultaneously performing a jaw thrust with one hand and squeezing the bag with the other. It is easy to hypoventilate due to a leak or to push down too hard and obstruct the airway. Bag-mask ventilation is better with two people (Figure 9.9). One person holds the face mask in place, using both hands and a jaw thrust, and the other squeezes the bag. The seal will be better, and the ventilation will be more effective and safer.

Excessive compression of the bag when used with a face mask can inflate the stomach, further reducing ventilation and greatly increasing the risk of regurgitation and aspiration. Avoid hyperventilation; a rate of 10 breaths min^{-1} is adequate.

Supraglottic airways during CPR

In comparison with bag-mask ventilation, use of supraglottic airways (SGAs) (e.g. i-gel) may enable more effective ventilation and reduce the risk of gastric inflation. Without adequate training and experience, the incidence of complications associated with attempted tracheal intubation is unacceptably high. Unrecognised oesophageal intubation is disastrous, and prolonged attempts at tracheal intubation are harmful: the pause in chest compressions during this time will severely compromise coronary and cerebral perfusion. Alternative airway devices should be used by all clinicians who are not skilled in tracheal intubation. If attempted tracheal intubation by those highly skilled in the technique has failed, alternative airway devices should be used.

Supraglottic airways sit above the larynx and are easier to insert than a tracheal tube. They can generally be inserted without having to stop chest compressions.

i-gel airway

The i-gel has a cuff made of jelly-like material and does not require inflation. The stem of the i-gel incorporates a bite block and a narrow oesophageal drain tube that allows a gastric tube to be passed through it (Figure 9.10). It is easy to insert without stopping CPR, requires only minimal training and forms a good laryngeal seal.

The ease of insertion of the i-gel and its favourable leak pressure make it very attractive as a resuscitation airway device for those inexperienced in tracheal intubation. Use of the i-gel during cardiac arrest has now been reported extensively, and it is in widespread use in the UK for both in-hospital and out-of-hospital cardiac arrest.

Technique for insertion of an i-gel

1. Ensure that the airway is clear of foreign bodies prior to insertion of the i-gel.
2. Try to maintain chest compressions throughout the insertion attempt; if it is necessary to stop chest compressions during the insertion attempt, limit this pause in chest compressions to a maximum of 5 s.
3. Select an appropriately sized i-gel: a size 4 (50–90 kg) will function well in most adults, although small adults (30–60 kg) may require a size 3, and large adults (> 90 kg) may require a size 5.
4. Lubricate the back, sides and front of the i-gel cuff with a thin layer of lubricant.
5. Grasp the lubricated i-gel firmly along the integral bite block. Position the device so that the i-gel cuff outlet is facing towards the chin of the patient.
6. Ensure the patient is in the 'sniffing the morning air' position with head extended and neck flexed. Gently press the chin down to open the mouth before inserting the i-gel.
7. Introduce the leading soft tip into the mouth of the patient in a direction towards the hard palate (Figure 9.11).
8. Do not apply excessive force to the device during insertion. It is not normally necessary to insert fingers or thumbs into the patient's mouth when inserting the i-gel. If there is early resistance during insertion, have an assistant apply a jaw thrust or gently rotate the i-gel.
9. Glide the i-gel downwards and backwards along the hard palate with a continuous but gentle push until a definitive resistance is felt.
10. At this point, the tip of the airway should be located at the upper oesophageal opening, and the cuff should be located against the larynx. The incisors should rest on the integral bite block.

Figure 9.11 Insertion of an i-gel during CPR

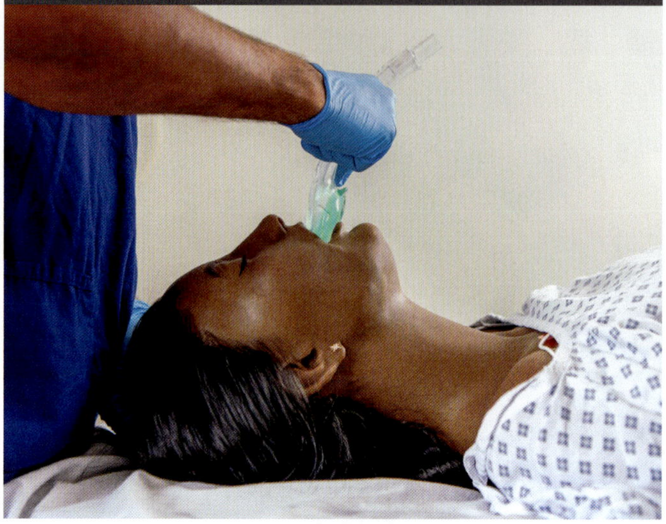

11. A horizontal line at the middle of the integral bite-block represents the approximate position of the teeth when the i-gel is positioned correctly. However, this line is only a guide – there is considerable variation in its location relative to the incisors. In short patients, this line may be at least 1 cm higher than the teeth, even when correctly positioned. In tall patients, the line may not be visible above the teeth.

Limitations of the i-gel

- In the presence of high airway resistance or poor lung compliance (pulmonary oedema, bronchospasm, chronic obstructive pulmonary disease), there is a risk of a significant leak around the cuff, causing hypoventilation. Most of the gas leaking around the cuff normally escapes through the patient's mouth, but some gastric inflation may occur.
- Uninterrupted chest compressions are likely to cause at least some gas leak from the i-gel cuff when ventilation is attempted. Attempt continuous compressions initially, but if gas leakage results in inadequate ventilation, pause compressions for ventilation using a compression to ventilation ratio of 30:2.
- There is a theoretical risk of aspiration of stomach contents because the i-gel does not sit within the larynx like a tracheal tube; however, this complication is rarely documented in clinical practice.
- If the patient is not deeply unconscious, insertion of the i-gel may cause coughing, straining or laryngeal spasm. This will not occur in patients in cardiorespiratory arrest.
- If an adequate airway is not achieved, withdraw the i-gel and attempt reinsertion, ensuring a good alignment of the head and neck.
- If satisfactory ventilation is not achieved after repositioning, remove the i-gel and use the 2-person BVM technique.

09 SUMMARY LEARNING

Airway management and ventilation are essential parts of cardiopulmonary resuscitation.

Airway obstruction can usually be relieved with simple techniques.

Simple adjuncts make airway management more effective and acceptable.

SGAs are an acceptable alternative to tracheal intubation and should be inserted by staff who have had adequate training.

TEST YOURSELF QUESTIONS

1. What are the signs of severe airway obstruction?
2. How do you size an oropharyngeal (Guedel) airway?
3. At what rate should you ventilate the lungs of a patient during cardiac arrest?

Further reading

Drennan IR, Greif R, Bray JE, et al., on behalf of the ILCOR Advanced Life Support Task Force. 2025 International Consensus on Cardiopulmonary Resuscitation and Emergency Cardiovascular Care Science With Treatment Recommendations. Advanced Life Support. ILCOR, 2025. In print.

Soar J, Böttiger B, Carli P, et al. European Resuscitation Council Guidelines 2025: Advanced Life Support. Resuscitation. 2025.In print.

My key take-home messages from this chapter are:

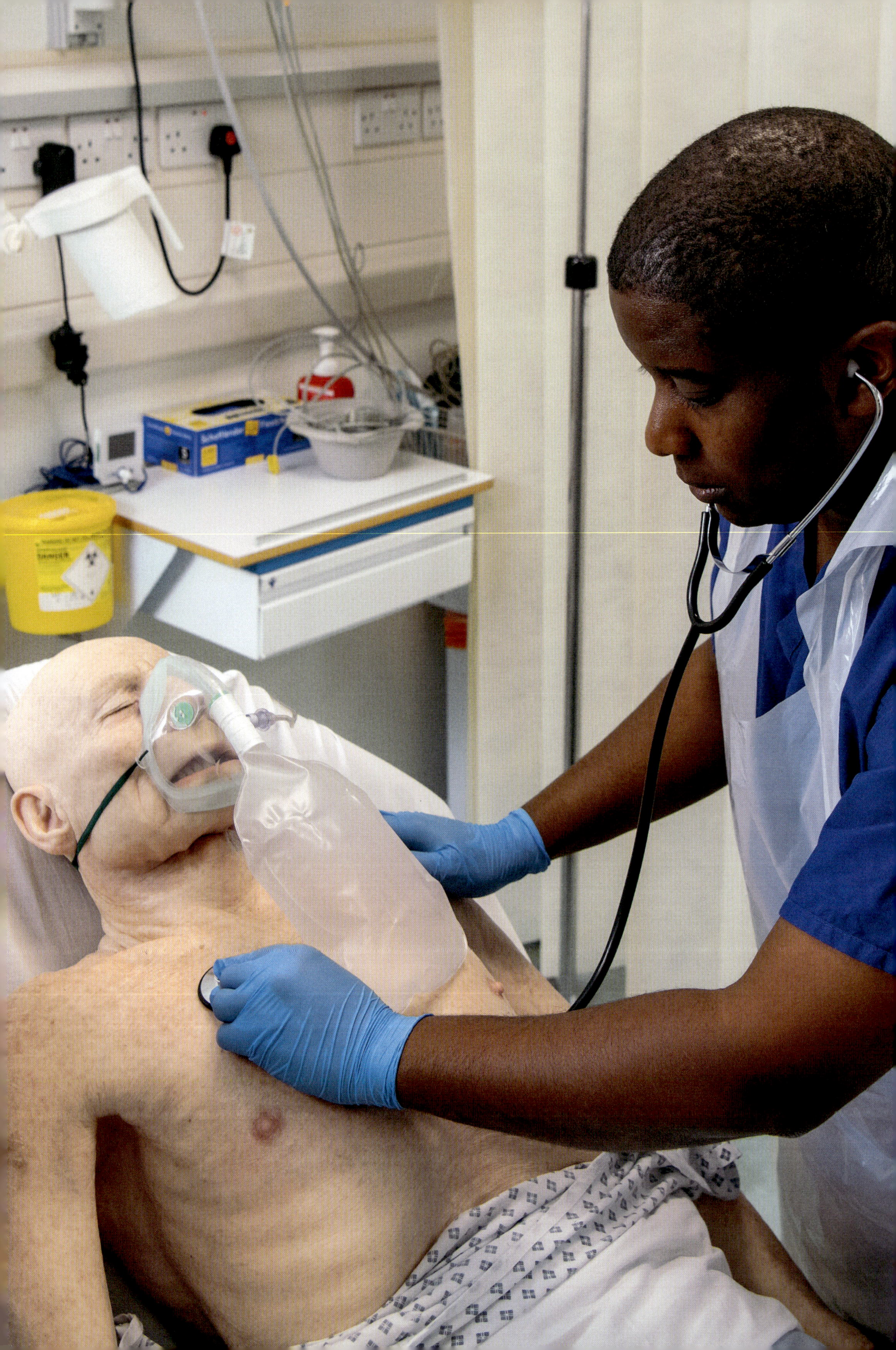

10 Post-resuscitation care

In this chapter

The post-cardiac arrest syndrome

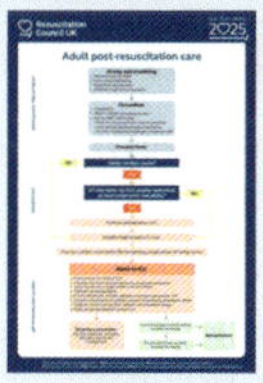

The adult post-resuscitation care algorithm

Optimising organ function

The learning outcomes will enable you to:

Understand the need for continued resuscitation after return of spontaneous circulation

Understand the post-cardiac arrest syndrome

Facilitate transfer of the patient safely

Introduction

Immediate Life Support (ILS) skills may be successful before expert help arrives. Return of spontaneous circulation (ROSC) is an important first step, but the ultimate goal of resuscitation is to return the patient to a state of normal cerebral function and to establish and maintain a stable cardiac rhythm and normal haemodynamic function.

The post-resuscitation care algorithm (Figure 10.2) shows the key steps for a successful outcome.

Many of the interventions are complex and require specialist help; they are provided here as an overview of the topic.

ILS providers only need to know the immediate steps to take, and ensure that help been called, so that the patient receives appropriate treatment.

The quality of treatment provided in this post-resuscitation phase, the final link in the Chain of Survival, significantly influences the patient's ultimate outcome. The post-resuscitation phase begins at the location where ROSC is achieved. Once stabilised, in the out-of-hospital setting, the patient should be conveyed to an appropriate receiving facility with a pre-alert call. In hospital, transfer the patient to the most appopriate high-care (e.g. intensive care unit (ICU), coronary care unit (CCU)) for further treatment.

The post-cardiac arrest syndrome

The post-cardiac arrest syndrome comprises:

- post-cardiac arrest brain injury
- post-cardiac arrest myocardial dysfunction
- systemic ischaemia/reperfusion response
- persistent precipitating pathology.

The severity of this syndrome will vary with the duration and cause of cardiac arrest. It may not occur at all if the cardiac arrest is brief.

- Post-cardiac arrest brain injury manifests as coma, seizures, myoclonus, varying degrees of neurological dysfunction and brain death.
- Significant myocardial dysfunction is common after cardiac arrest but typically recovers by 2–3 days.
- The whole-body ischaemia/reperfusion that occurs with resuscitation from cardiac arrest activates immunological and coagulation pathways, contributing to multiple organ failure and increasing the risk of infection.
- The persistent precipitating pathology is what caused the cardiac arrest in the first place. For example, if the patient had a myocardial infarction, this would have an impact on the heart's function.
- The post-cardiac arrest syndrome has many features in common with sepsis, including intravascular volume depletion and vasodilation.

Figure 10.1 The ABCDE assessment to post-resuscitation care

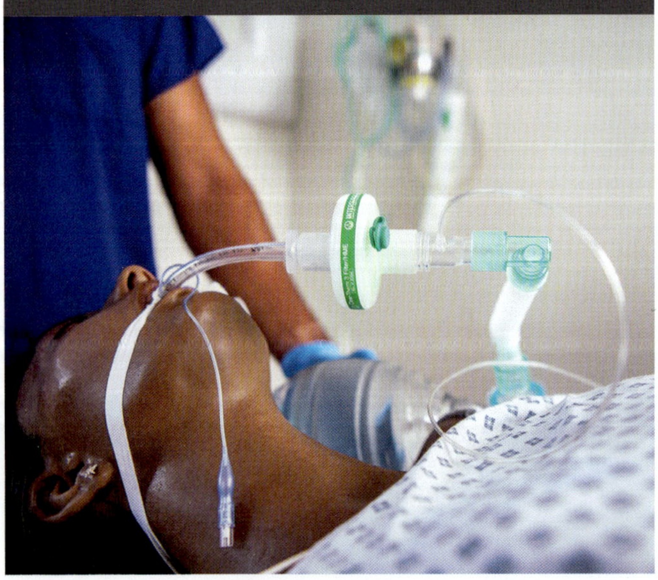

Continued resuscitation

In the immediate post-resuscitation phase, treat the patient by following the ABCDE assessment (Figure 10.2).

A B C D E

A = Airway and B = Breathing

Aim: to ensure a clear airway, adequate oxygenation and ventilation.

Patients who have had a brief period of cardiac arrest that responded immediately to appropriate treatment (e.g. witnessed ventricular fibrillation (VF) or pulseless ventricular tachycardia (pVT) reverting to sinus rhythm after early defibrillation) may achieve an immediate return of normal cerebral function. These patients do not require tracheal intubation and ventilation but should be given oxygen by face mask if needed to maintain a normal arterial oxygen saturation. Other patients may not be immediately neurologically normal, even after a rapid, successful resuscitation. Hypoxia and hypercapnia both increase the likelihood of a further cardiac arrest and can cause secondary brain injury.

Studies suggest that high levels of oxygen in the blood (hyperoxaemia) after resuscitation from cardiac arrest can also be harmful. As soon as arterial blood oxygen saturation can be monitored reliably (by blood gas analysis and/or pulse oximetry (SpO_2)), titrate the inspired oxygen concentration to maintain the arterial blood oxygen saturation in the range of 94–98%. Consider tracheal intubation, sedation and controlled ventilation in patients with obtunded cerebral function. This requires expert help. The patient's lungs are ventilated, aiming to achieve a normal arterial blood carbon dioxide concentration ($PaCO_2$).

Examine the patient's chest and look for symmetrical chest movement. Listen to ensure that the breath sounds are equal on both sides. A tracheal tube that has been inserted too far will tend to go down the right main bronchus and fail to ventilate the left lung. If ribs have been fractured during chest compression, there may be a pneumothorax (reduced or absent breath sounds) or a flail segment. Listen for evidence of pulmonary oedema or pulmonary aspiration of gastric contents. Insert a gastric tube – this will decompress the stomach following bag-mask ventilation, prevent splinting of the diaphragm, and enable drainage of gastric contents.

If the intubated patient regains consciousness soon after ROSC, is cooperative and breathing normally, consider immediate extubation: coughing on the tracheal tube may provoke arrhythmias and/or hypertension. If immediate or early extubation is not possible, sedate the patient to ensure the tracheal tube is tolerated, and provide ventilatory support.

Adult post-resuscitation care

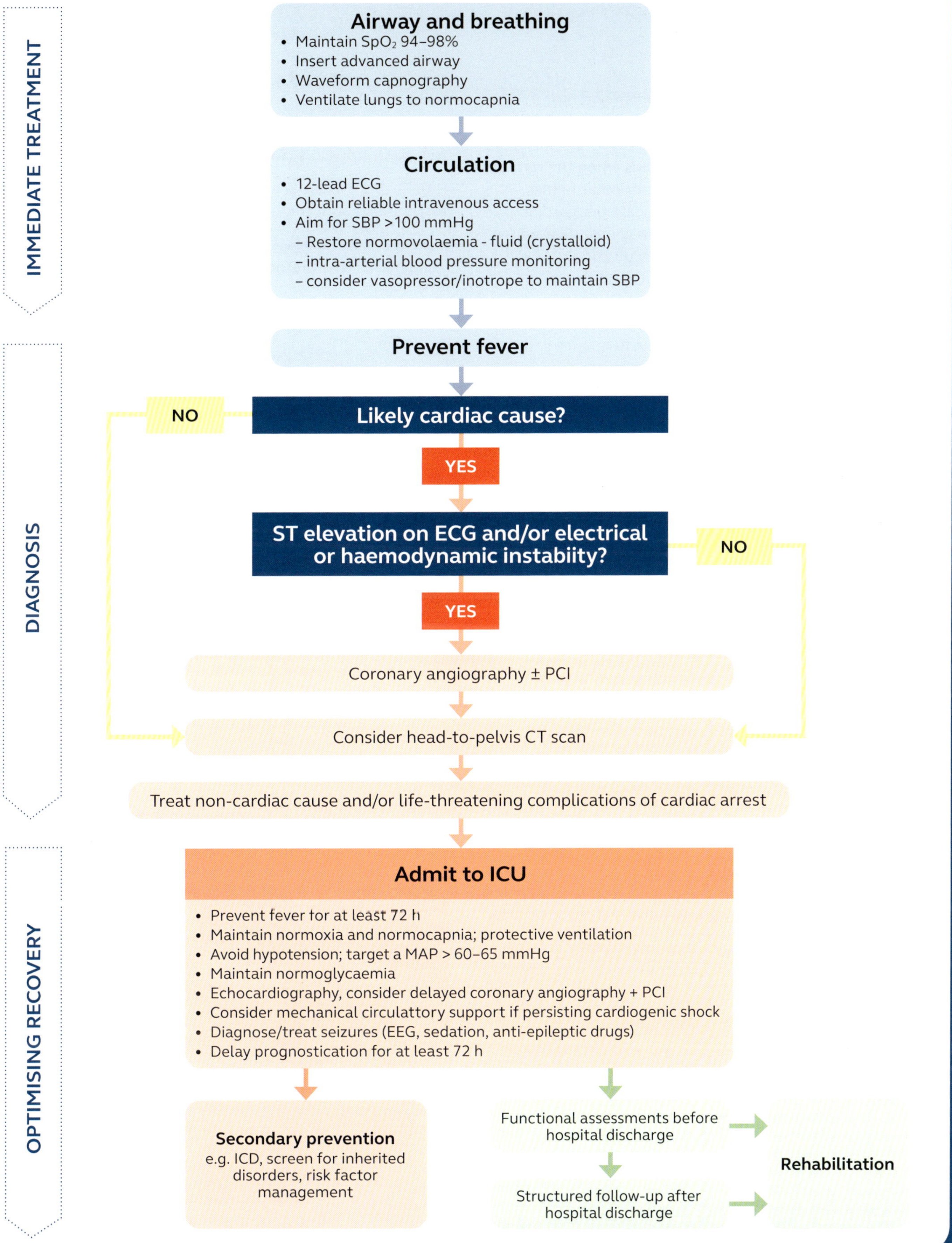

Figure 10.2 Adult post-resuscitation care algorithm – **SBP** systolic blood pressure, **PCI** percutaneous coronary intervention, **ICU** Intensive care unit, **MAP** mean arterial pressure, **EEG** electroencephalography, **ICD** implanted cardioverter defibrillator

C = Circulation

Aim: the maintenance of normal sinus rhythm and a cardiac output adequate for perfusion of vital organs.

Cardiac rhythm and blood pressure are likely to be unstable following a cardiac arrest. Continuous ECG monitoring is essential. Record the pulse and blood pressure, and assess peripheral perfusion: warm, perfused fingers with a rapid capillary refill usually imply adequate perfusion. Grossly distended neck veins when the patient is semi-upright may indicate right ventricular failure, but in rare cases, they could also indicate pericardial tamponade. Left ventricular failure may be indicated by fine inspiratory crackles heard on auscultation of the lungs, and the production of pink frothy sputum. If the facility for direct continuous arterial blood pressure monitoring is available, insert an arterial cannula to enable reliable monitoring during transfer. Once in a high-care area, the use of non-invasive cardiac output monitoring devices is useful.

Infusion of fluids may be required to increase right heart filling pressures, or conversely, diuretics and vasodilators may be needed to treat left ventricular failure.

Record a 12-lead ECG as soon as possible. Acute ST-segment elevation or new left bundle branch block in a patient with a typical history of acute myocardial infarction is an indication for treatment to try to re-open an occluded coronary artery (reperfusion therapy). This is usually achieved by emergency percutaneous coronary intervention (PCI). Services should aim to achieve a 'call-to-balloon' time (i.e. time from call for help to attempted re-opening of the culprit artery) of < 120 minutes whenever possible. Consider fibrinolytic therapy if this is not possible. Cardiopulmonary resuscitation, even if prolonged, is not a contraindication to fibrinolytic therapy.

In post-resuscitation patients, chest pain and/or ST-elevation are relatively poor predictors of acute coronary occlusion; for this reason, primary PCI should be considered in all post-resuscitation patients who are suspected of having coronary artery disease as the cause of their arrest, even if they are sedated and mechanically ventilated.

D = Disability

Aim: to evaluate the neurological function.

Although it may not be of immediate significance to the patient's management, assess neurological function rapidly and record the Glasgow Coma Scale score (GCS) (Table 10.1).

The maximum score possible is 15;
the minimum score possible is 3.

Re-check the patient's glucose and record pupillary response to light (Figure 10.2).

Table 10.1 The Glasgow Coma Scale

Eye opening	Spontaneously	4
	To speech	3
	To pain	2
	Nil	1
Verbal	Oriented	5
	Confused	4
	Inappropriate words	3
	Incomprehensible sounds	2
	Nil	1
Best motor response	Obeys commands	6
	Localises	5
	Normal flexion	4
	Abnormal flexion	3
	Extension	2
	Nil	1

Figure 10.2 Pupillary response to light

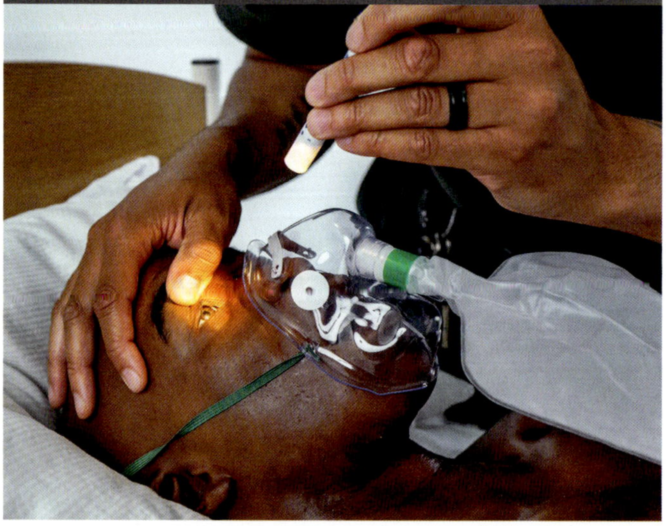

E = Exposure

Aim: to ensure that cardiac arrest has not been associated with other medical or surgical conditions requiring immediate treatment.

Although cardiac arrest is caused frequently by primary cardiac disease, other precipitating conditions must be excluded, particularly in-hospital patients (e.g. massive blood loss, respiratory failure, pulmonary embolism).

Assess the other body systems rapidly so that further resuscitation is appropriate for the patient's needs. To examine the patient properly, full exposure of the body may be necessary.

Provide continuous monitoring of core temperature in patients who remain comatose after ROSC from cardiac arrest and actively prevent fever (> 37.7°C) for at least 72 hours. Temperature control can be achieved by exposing the patient, using anti-pyretic drugs, or if this is insufficient, by using a cooling device with a target temperature of 37.5°C.

Further assessment

Patient history

Aim: to establish the patient's state of health and regular drug therapy before the cardiac arrest.

Obtain a comprehensive history as quickly as possible. Those involved in caring for the patient immediately before the cardiac arrest may be able to provide assistance (e.g. paramedics, ward staff, and relatives (Figure 10.3).

Ask specifically about symptoms of cardiac disease.

If primary cardiac disease seems unlikely, consider other causes of cardiac arrest (e.g. drug overdose, subarachnoid haemorrhage).

Make a note of any delay before the start of resuscitation and the duration of the resuscitation; this may have prognostic significance, although it is generally unreliable and should not be used alone to predict outcome.

The patient's baseline physiological reserve (before the cardiac arrest) is one of the most important factors taken into consideration by the ICU team when determining whether prolonged multiple organ support is appropriate.

Figure 10.3 Obtaining a history from a relative

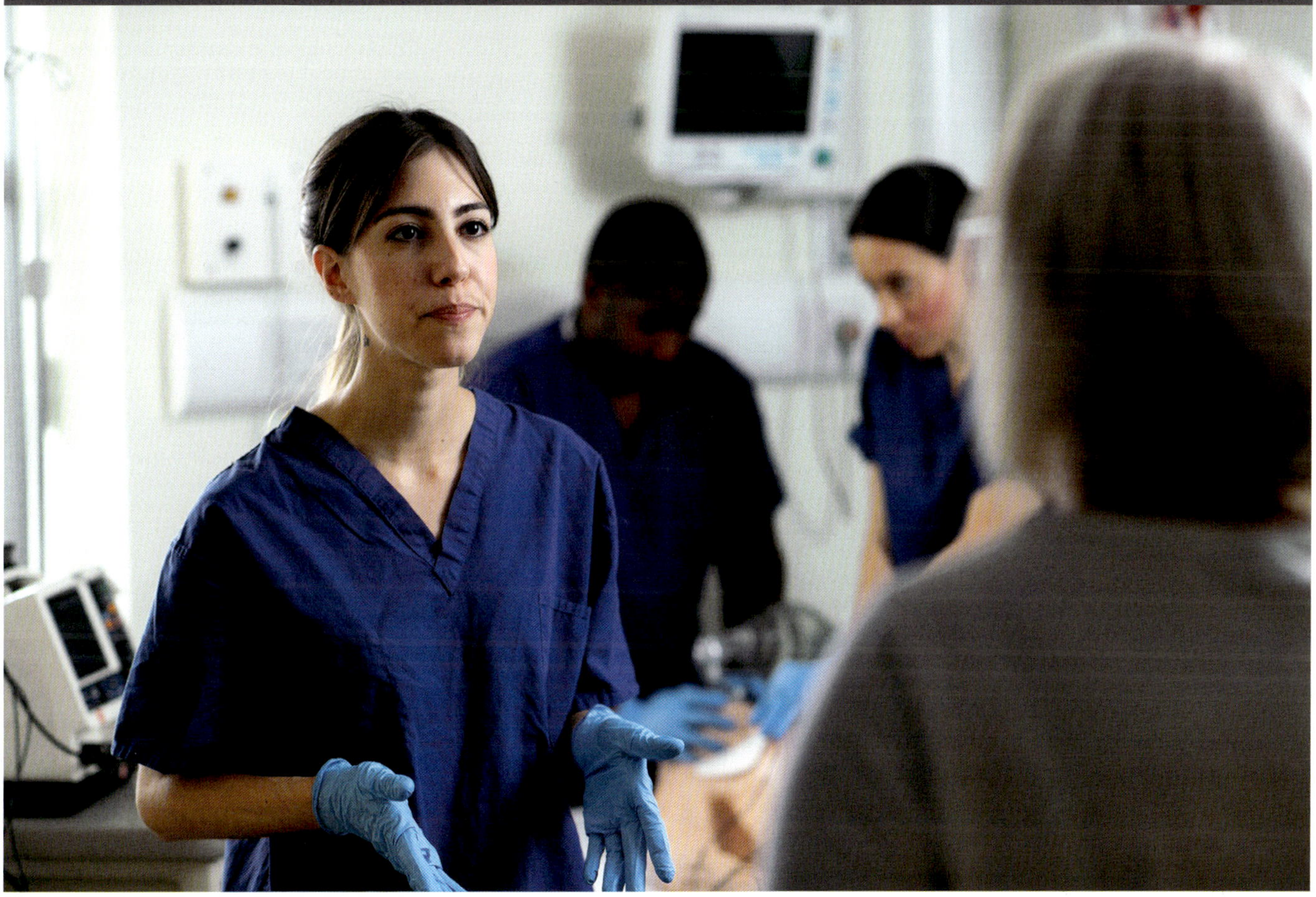

Monitoring

Aim: to enable continuous assessment of vital organ function and to identify trends.

Continuous monitoring of ECG, arterial blood pressures, respiratory rate, pulse oximetry, capnography, core temperature and urinary output is essential to detect changes during the period of instability that follows resuscitation from cardiac arrest. Monitor the effects of medical interventions (e.g. assisted ventilation, diuretic therapy) continuously. This will require expert help.

Investigations

Aim: to undertake appropriate and urgent investigations.

Several physiological variables may be abnormal immediately after a cardiac arrest, and urgent biochemical and cardiological investigations should be undertaken (Table 10.2).

Patient transfer

Aim: to transfer the patient safely between the site of resuscitation and a place of definitive care.

Following the period of initial post-resuscitation care and stabilisation, the patient will need to be transferred to an appropriate critical care setting (e.g. ICU or CCU). Out-of-hospital teams will need to convey to an appropriate receiving hospital unit such as the emergency department or PCI centre. The decision to transfer should be made only after discussion with senior members of the admitting team. Handover care using SBARD or RSVP (Table 4.1). Continue all established monitoring during the transfer and secure all cannulae, catheters, tubes and drains. Conduct a full reassessment immediately before transferring the patient. Ensure that the portable suction apparatus, oxygen supply, defibrillator, and monitor accompany the patient and transfer team.

The transfer team should comprise individuals capable of monitoring the patient and responding appropriately to any changes in the patient's condition, including a further cardiac arrest. The Faculty of Intensive Care Medicine (FICM) and the Intensive Care Society (UK) have published guidelines for the transport of critically ill adults. These outline the requirements for equipment and personnel when transferring critically ill patients.

Table 10.2 Investigations after restoration of circulation

Full blood count	To exclude anaemia as a contributor to myocardial ischaemia and provide baseline values
Biochemistry	To assess renal function
	To assess electrolyte concentrations (K^+, Mg^{2+}, and Ca^{2+})
	To ensure normoglycaemia
	To commence serial cardiac troponin measurements
	To provide baseline values
12-lead ECG	To record cardiac rhythm
	To look for evidence of acute coronary syndrome
	To look for evidence of old myocardial infarction
	To provide a baseline record
Chest radiograph	To establish the position of tracheal tube, a gastric tube, and/or a central venous catheter
	To check for evidence of pulmonary oedema
	To check for evidence of pulmonary aspiration
	To exclude pneumothorax
	To assess cardiac contour (accurate assessment of heart size requires standard PA erect radiograph – not always practicable in the post-resuscitation situation)
Arterial blood gases	To ensure adequacy of ventilation and oxygenation
	To ensure correction of acid/base imbalance
Echocardiography	To identify contributing causes to cardiac arrest
	To assess LV and RV structure and function

10 SUMMARY LEARNING

After cardiac arrest, return of spontaneous circulation is just the first stage in a continuum of resuscitation.

The quality of post-resuscitation care will significantly influence the patient's final outcome.

These patients require appropriate monitoring, safe transfer to a critical care environment, and continued organ support.

The post-cardiac arrest syndrome comprises post-cardiac arrest brain injury, post-cardiac arrest myocardial dysfunction, the systemic ischaemia/ reperfusion response, and persistence of precipitating pathology.

TEST YOURSELF QUESTIONS

1. What blood oxygen saturation should be targeted for post-cardiac arrest patients?
2. What is the lowest possible score on the Glasgow Coma Score (GCS)?

Further reading

Drennan IR, Greif R, Bray JE, et al., on behalf of the ILCOR Advanced Life Support Task Force. 2025 International Consensus on Cardiopulmonary Resuscitation and Emergency Cardiovascular Care Science With Treatment Recommendations. Advanced Life Support. ILCOR, 2025. In print.

Guidance On: The Transfer Of The Critically Ill Adult. 2019. www.ficm.ac.uk or www.ics.ac.uk

Nolan JP, Sandroni C, Cariou, A et al. European Resuscitation Council and European Society of Intensive Care Medicine Guidelines 2025: Post-resuscitation care. Resuscitation. 2025. In print.

Nolan JP, Neumar RW, Adrie C, et al. Post-cardiac arrest syndrome: epidemiology, pathophysiology, treatment, and prognostication. A Scientific Statement from the International Liaison Committee on Resuscitation; the American Heart Association Emergency Cardiovascular Care Committee; the Council on Cardiovascular Surgery and Anesthesia; the Council on Cardiopulmonary, Perioperative, and Critical Care; the Council on Clinical Cardiology; the Council on Stroke. Resuscitation 2008;79:350-79.

Nolan JP, Sandroni C, Andersen LW, Böttiger BW, Cariou A, Cronberg T, Friberg H, Genbrugge C, Lilja G, Morley PT, Nikolaou N, Olasveengen TM, Skrifvars MB, Taccone FS, Soar J. ERC-ESICM guidelines on temperature control after cardiac arrest in adults. Resuscitation. 2022 Mar;172:229-236.

Soar J, Böttiger B, Carli P, et al. European Resuscitation Council Guidelines 2025: Advanced Life Support. Resuscitation. 2025.In print.

My key take-home messages from this chapter are:

Appendix A
Drugs commonly used during the treatment of cardiac arrest

Drug			
Adrenaline	**Shockable (VF/pVT)** **Dose:** **1 mg in 10 mL (1:10 000) IV/IO** Given after the 3rd cycle, once compressions have been resumed Repeated every 3–5 min (alternate cycles) Given without interrupting chest compressions	**Non-Shockable (PEA/Asystole)** **Dose:** **1 mg in 10 mL (1:10 000) IV/IO** Given as soon as circulatory access is obtained Repeated every 3–5 min (alternate cycles) Given without interrupting chest compressions	Adrenaline has been the primary sympathomimetic drug for the management of cardiac arrest for over 50 years. Its alpha-adrenergic effects cause systemic vasoconstriction, which increases coronary and cerebral perfusion pressures. The beta-adrenergic actions of adrenaline (inotropic, chronotropic) may increase coronary and cerebral blood flow, but concomitant increases in myocardial oxygen consumption and ectopic ventricular arrhythmias (particularly in the presence of acidaemia), transient hypoxaemia because of pulmonary arteriovenous shunting, impaired microcirculation, and increased post-cardiac arrest myocardial dysfunction may offset these benefits. Use of adrenaline increases ROSC and the number of survivors with both a favourable and poor neurological outcome. The potential benefit may be greater when adrenaline is given early for cardiac arrest with a non-shockable rhythm.
Amiodarone	**Shockable (VF/pVT)** **Dose:** **300 mg bolus IV/IO diluted in 5% dextrose (or other suitable solvent) to a volume of 20 mL** Given during chest compressions after three defibrillation attempts Further dose of 150 mg if VF/pVT persists after five defibrillation attempts	**Non-Shockable (PEA/Asystole)** **Not indicated for PEA or asystole**	Amiodarone is a membrane-stabilising anti-arrhythmic drug that increases the duration of the action potential and refractory period in atrial and ventricular myocardium. Atrioventricular conduction is slowed, and a similar effect is seen with accessory pathways. Amiodarone has a mild negative inotropic action and causes peripheral vasodilation through non-competitive alpha-blocking effects. Amiodarone may improve short-term survival, especially when it is given early after the onset of cardiac arrest. Amiodarone should be flushed with 0.9% sodium chloride or 5% dextrose.
Fluids	**Infuse fluids rapidly if hypovolaemia is suspected.** Use sodium chloride 0.9%, or balanced crystalloid (e.g. Hartmann's solution, Ringer's lactate) or blood for major haemorrhage where necessary. Avoid dextrose, which is redistributed away from the intravascular space rapidly and causes hyperglycaemia, which may worsen neurological outcome and survival after cardiac arrest. Give fluids during a cardiac arrest only if there is evidence of hypovolaemia.		

Appendix B
Pulse oximetry and oxygen therapy

Pulse oximetry

Pulse oximetry is a vital adjunct to the assessment of hypoxaemia. Clinical recognition of decreased arterial oxygen saturation is subjective and unreliable; a person may not appear to be cyanosed until their arterial oxygen saturation is as low as 80–85%. Pulse oximeters work by detecting changes in oxygenated haemoglobin in the blood. They do this by shining light through the tissue, but they depend on having a reasonable circulation to the area of the body where the probe is attached. Use an appropriate pulse oximeter probe to monitor oxygen saturations; for example, a finger probe should not be used on an ear (or vice versa).

Pulse oximeters often provide an audible tone related to the SpO_2 value, with a decreasing tone reflecting increasing hypoxaemia. This can be helpful, since you can detect changes in SpO_2 just by listening, even if you aren't looking at the screen.

Some pulse oximeters, particularly those used in areas such as the emergency department (ED), intensive care unit (ICU), operating room, or ambulance services, also display a waveform. This gives useful information about the quality of the signal the system is measuring. A poor signal may indicate low blood pressure or poor tissue perfusion, and may also mean that the SpO_2 measurement is inaccurate.

Limitations of pulse oximetry

There are several potential sources of error with pulse oximetry:

- Presence of other haemoglobins: carboxyhaemoglobin (carbon monoxide poisoning), methaemoglobin (congenital or acquired), and sickling red cells (sickle cell disease).
- Surgical and imaging dyes (e.g. methylene blue) can cause falsely low saturation readings.
- Nail varnish (especially blue, black and green).
- High-ambient light levels (fluorescent and xenon lamps).
- Motion artefact.

Reduced pulse volume:

- hypotension
- low cardiac output
- vasoconstriction
- hypothermia.

Pulse oximeters are not affected by:

- anaemia (reduced haemoglobin)
- jaundice (hyperbilirubinaemia).

Black and brown skin may lead to an overestimation of the oxygen saturation value; therefore, consider both relative changes in an individual patient's readings and the numerical result.

Pulse oximetry does not provide a reliable signal during CPR. The blood oxygen saturations are measured only where the system can detect a pulse. If blood oxygen saturations are completely unrecordable, this is more likely to reflect a 'C' problem than a 'B' problem.

Targeted oxygen therapy

Target SpO_2 to 94–98% for all patients (unless type II respiratory failure confirmed by arterial blood gas analysis). Initially, use a mask with a reservoir (a non-rebreather mask) at 15 L min^{-1}. Titrate according to 94–98% (or 88–92% in confirmed type II respiratory failure) once an accurate SpO_2 reading is achieved with an appropriately fitted device (e.g. venturi, nasal cannulae).

Special clinical situations

Patients with respiratory failure

Respiratory failure can be divided into two groups:

Type I Respiratory Failure:
low PaO_2 (< 8 kPa), normal $PaCO_2$ (< 7 kPa)

In these patients, it is safe to initially administer a high concentration of oxygen with the goal of returning their PaO_2 to normal levels. Once clinically stable, the inspired oxygen concentration can then be adjusted to maintain an SpO_2 of 94–98%.

Type II Respiratory Failure:
low PaO_2 (< 8 kPa), increased $PaCO_2$ (> 7 kPa).

This is often described as hypercapnic respiratory failure and is often caused by COPD. If given excessive oxygen, these patients may develop worsening respiratory failure with further increases in $PaCO_2$ and the development of a respiratory acidosis. If unchecked, this will eventually lead to unconsciousness and respiratory and/or cardiac arrest.

The target oxygen saturation in this at-risk population is 88–92%. However, when critically ill and their arterial blood oxygen saturation is unknown, give these patients high-flow oxygen initially, then analyse the arterial blood gases and use the results to adjust the inspired oxygen concentration. When the patient is clinically stable and a reliable pulse oximetry reading is obtained, adjust the inspired oxygen concentration to maintain an SpO_2 of 88–92%. **Administering oxygen to these patients is not inherently dangerous, but failing to monitor them carefully can be.** If there is a concern that a patient may have Type II respiratory failure and is receiving oxygen therapy, ensure that frequent observations are conducted to monitor their condition. Initially, you may need to take frequent ABG samples. If their CO_2 levels are rising, then they may be receiving too much oxygen. Oxygen delivery may need to be reviewed, and the oxygen concentration adjusted accordingly. Assistance may be needed from respiratory physicians or intensive care, as the patient may require ventilatory support.

Patients with acute coronary syndrome

In patients with a myocardial infarction or an acute coronary syndrome, and who are not critically or seriously ill, aim to maintain an SpO_2 of 94–98% (or 88–92% if the patient is also at risk of hypercapnic respiratory failure). This may be achievable **without** the need for supplementary oxygen.

Appendix C
Asthma

From British Thoracic Society/Scottish Intercollegiate Guidelines Network Guideline on the Management of Asthma

www.brit-thoracic.org.uk

Levels of severity of acute asthma attacks in adults

Asthma severity	Clinical signs/measurements:	Investigations:
Near-fatal asthma	• Raised $PaCO_2$ **and/or** • mechanical ventilation with raised inflation pressures	
Life-threatening asthma	**Any ONE of the following in a patient with severe asthma:** • PEF < 33% of best or predicted value • SpO_2 < 92% • Silent chest, cyanosis, or poor respiratory effort • Arrhythmia or hypotension • Exhaustion, altered consciousness	If a patient has any life-threatening features, measure arterial blood gases. No other investigations are needed for immediate management. Blood gas markers of a life-threatening attack: • 'Normal' (4.6–6 kPa, 35–45 mmHg) $PaCO_2$ • Severe hypoxia: PaO_2 < 8 kPa (60 mmHg) irrespective of treatment with oxygen • A low pH (or high H^+). Caution: Patients with severe or life-threatening attacks may not be distressed and may not have all these abnormalities. The presence of any should alert the doctor.
Acute severe asthma	**Any ONE of:** • PEF 33–50% of best or predicted value • Respiratory rate ≥ 25 min^{-1} • Heart rate ≥ 110 min^{-1} • Inability to complete sentences in one breath	
Moderate acute asthma	• Increasing symptoms • PEF > 50–75% of best or predicted value • SpO_2 ≥ 92% • Speech normal • Respiration < 25 breaths min^{-1} • Pulse < 110 beats min^{-1} • No features of acute severe asthma	

SpO_2 – oxygen saturation measured by a pulse oximeter

PaO_2 – partial arterial pressure of oxygen

kPa – kilopascals

$PaCO_2$ – partial arterial pressure of carbon dioxide

Further information

British Thoracic Society/Scottish Intercollegiate Guidelines Network Guideline Asthma pathway (BTS, NICE, SIGN) [SIGN 244] 2024. www.brit-thoracic.org.uk

Appendix D
Anaphylaxis algorithm

Anaphylaxis

Anaphylaxis?

A = Airway B = Breathing C = Circulation D = Disability E = Exposure

Diagnosis – look for:
- Sudden onset of Airway and/or Breathing and/or Circulation problems[1]
- And usually skin changes (e.g. itchy rash)

Call for HELP
Call resuscitation team or ambulance

- Remove trigger if possible (e.g. stop any infusion)
- Lie patient flat (with or without legs elevated)
  - A sitting position may make breathing easier
  - If pregnant, lie on left side

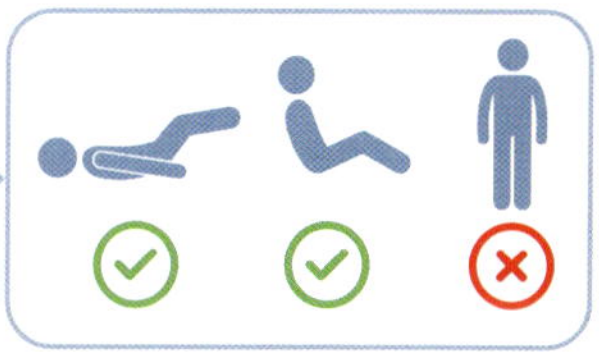

Give intramuscular (IM) adrenaline[2]

Inject at **anterolateral aspect** – middle third of the thigh

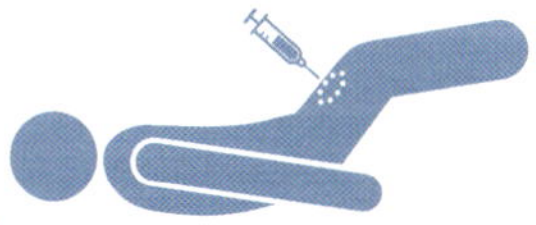

- Establish airway
- Give high flow oxygen
- Apply monitoring: pulse oximetry, ECG, blood pressure

If no response:
- Repeat IM adrenaline after 5 minutes
- IV fluid bolus[3]

If no improvement in Breathing or Circulation problems[1] despite TWO doses of IM adrenaline:
- Confirm resuscitation team or ambulance has been called
- Follow REFRACTORY ANAPHYLAXIS ALGORITHM

1. Life-threatening problems

Airway
Hoarse voice, stridor

Breathing
↑work of breathing, wheeze, fatigue, cyanosis, $SpO_2 < 94\%$

Circulation
Low blood pressure, signs of shock, confusion, reduced consciousness

2. Intramuscular (IM) adrenaline

Use adrenaline at 1 mg/mL (1:1000) concentration

Adult and child > 12 years:	500 micrograms IM (0.5 mL)
Child 6–12 years:	300 micrograms IM (0.3 mL)
Child 6 months to 6 years:	150 micrograms IM (0.15 mL)
Child < 6 months:	100–150 micrograms IM (0.1–0.15 mL)

The above doses are for IM injection **only**.
Intravenous adrenaline for anaphylaxis to be given **only by experienced specialists** in an appropriate setting.

3. IV fluid challenge

Use crystalloid

Adults:	500–1000 mL
Children:	10 mL/kg

Appendix E
Useful links

Become an RCUK ILS Instructor

Exceptional candidates may be identified by the faculty to become an ILS instructor. The Course Director and faculty must support the nomination and provide a detailed statement of support to RCUK.

To be successfully put forward as an Instructor Potential (IP), the candidate must be a statutory/ voluntary registered healthcare professional with at least two years post-qualification experience, work in an appropriate clinical setting, and be involved in resuscitation or resuscitation training as part of their work. Candidates must demonstrate excellent core knowledge of the course content, excellent and safe practical application of skills, and have exceptional communication skills.

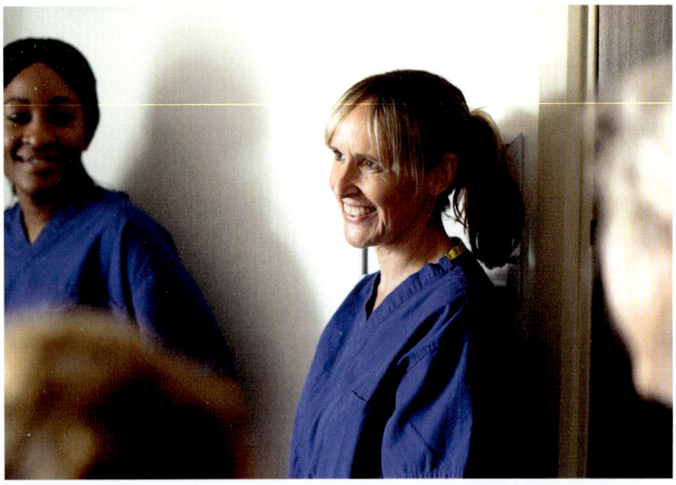

Potential instructors should be confident, flexible, adaptable, interactive, supportive and enthusiastic. If successfully nominated, the candidate would need to undertake an RCUK ILSi course and complete two supported supervised teaching practices as an Instructor Candidate (IC).

More information on ILSi can be accessed here: www.resus.org.uk/ training-courses/instructor-courses/ ilsi-immediate-life-support-instructor-course.

Benefits of becoming an instructor for RCUK

You will join the RCUK community of practice with opportunities for portfolio development and ongoing access to the latest research and resuscitation practices.

You will become a subject matter expert, and your instructor qualification will be recognised throughout the UK and Europe.

As an instructor, you'll be eligible to attend RCUK's popular Instructor Days, and you will also receive free RCUK Associate membership.

Being an active ILS instructor means you are also an ILS provider.

For more information on how you can become an RCUK ILS instructor, please speak to the Course Director before or on the day of your course.

Resuscitation Council UK Guidelines
Read all of the 2025 guidelines:
resus.org.uk/2025-guidelines

Lifesaver app
Teach lifesaving skills anytime, anywhere with our Lifesaver products
resus.org.uk/lifesaver

iResus app
Get RCUK guidelines on the go:
resus.org.uk/iresus

Become ResusReady
Help us map CPR training across the UK:
resus.org.uk/resusready

Resuscitation Council UK courses
See all of the courses available:
resus.org.uk/professional-training

Follow us on LinkedIn
linkedin.com/company/resuscounciluk

RCUK membership
Get involved and join our community:
resus.org.uk/membership

Like us on Facebook
facebook.com/ResuscitationCouncilUK

Index

Index

V

W

Notes

Notes

Notes